the essential five

a grown-up girl's handbook for everything

kate etue & recah theodosiou

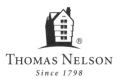

THOMAS NELSON
Since 1798

NASHVILLE   DALLAS   MEXICO CITY   RIO DE JANEIRO   BEIJING

Published in Nashville, Tennessee, by Thomas Nelson. Thomas Nelson is a registered trademark of Thomas Nelson, Inc.

Thomas Nelson, Inc. titles may be purchased in bulk for educational, business, fund-raising, or sales promotional use. For information, please e-mail SpecialMarkets@thomasnelson.com.

Kate Etue and Recah Theodosiou write courtesy of SNAP, LLC. For more information visit www.snaprepublic.com.

The discounts you will find in *The Essential Five* cannot be combined with any other discounts or promotions and are subject to change or cancellation at any time by the companies offering them.

Illustrations on section title pages by Anderson Thomas Design.

Page Design and other illustrations by Kay Meadows, Book & Graphic Design, Thomas Nelson, Inc., Nashville, Tennessee.

Cover Art by Anderson Thomas Design.

Quotes taken from *Friends*, *Gilmore Girls*, and *The OC* used by permission of Warner Bros. Entertainment Inc.

Library of Congress Cataloging-in-Publication Data

Etue, Kate.
    The essential five : the grown-up girl's handbook for everything /
Kate Etue and Recah Theodosiou.
      p. cm.
    Includes bibliographical references.
    ISBN 978-0-8499-1974-9 (pbk.)
    1. Women—Psychology. 2. Women—Conduct of life. I. Theodosiou,
Recah. II. Title. III. Title: Essential 5.
HQ1206.E895 2008
646.70082–dc22

                                    2007031223

Printed in the United States of America

08 09 10 11 RRD 6 5 4 3 2

A girl should be two things:
classy and fabulous.

—Coco Chanel

contents

Part One

Social Butterfly: Relationship Essentials

contents

Part Two

Classy and Fabulous: Lifestyle Essentials

contents

Part Three

Domestic Goddess: Home Essentials

contents

Part Four

Fetching and Fit: Body Essentials

contents

Part Five

Does It All: All the Other Essentials

acknowledgments

First things first: we're incredibly thankful to Debbie Wickwire, who came up with the idea for "this book of all these lists of five things" and thought to ask us to write it! Thanks to Adria Haley, Greg MacLachlan, Kay Meadows, and all the other hardworking folks at Nelson who did their part to make sure the book became a reality, including all the "grown-up" girls who unselfishly gave their time and ideas—Debbie Nichols, Jennifer McNeil, Jennifer Day, Kristi Johnson, Brandi Lewis, and Sally Hofmann. And, of course, thanks to David Moberg and Joey Paul for green-lighting the project and giving us a chance to become authors and not just editors!

But yikes, once the project was approved, we actually had to write the thing! We definitely want to thank each other—neither one of us could have written this alone, and it's been fantastic to share the experiences of each bringing a baby and this book into the world at the same time. And others helped so much as well. We want to mention everyone who gave us advice on our lists, specifically Suzanne Williams, Cathy Sullivan, Randy Draughon, Susan Kelton, Rhonda Hogan, Tiffany Etue, George Jones, Alex Fraser, John Anderson, Arwen Bowman, Lucille Bowman, and Stephanie Theodosiou, and especially those who read the whole thing and told us what parts were completely terrible: Meg Ashworth, Ellen Anderson, Katheryn Hutcheson, Natalie Fraser, and Susan Trotman.

We truly believe that this book would not be the future Pulitzer prize-winning, *New York Times* best-selling book it's destined to become if it weren't for Lori Jones, who we would have demanded be hired as our copyeditor if our editors hadn't so readily agreed that she *must* be the one to work on it as well. She's very good at what she does—and it gave us an excuse to write off all our lunches together!

acknowledgments

We should definitely mention our families and especially our husbands— Todd Etue and Marc Theodosiou. Not only do we love them; they were actually a tremendous help in writing this book. They made some really insightful (and quite funny) contributions to the manuscript. So thanks, guys! And Kate would like to mention her little boy, Grey. Although he'll just be turning two when we finish the book and hasn't contributed much in the way of actual feedback, he's given both of us ideas for material to write through his sweet but frequently mischievous behavior!

In an effort to avoid sounding like an Oscar acceptance speech gone on way too long (we can hear the music starting up now . . .), we'll leave it at that. There are dozens more people we could thank, but we'll just take the rest of the credit for ourselves!

introduction

You're fabulous and fun loving. Probably overcommitted. Definitely all about enjoying life. But your busy social calendar and fast-paced career life, or the myriad responsibilities of home life and charity projects, can become overwhelming—and even boring. You need to simplify!

Wouldn't it be simpler if we all just stuck to an unwritten rule of "five." Five ingredients. Five steps. Five people to contact. Five items to keep on hand. No more endless explanations or complicated systems. Five is so much more manageable, so much more doable.

Well, that's our goal for you in this book. These are the "essential five" things you need to know . . . about everything serious and fun, important and not! Need to get rid of that annoying "pest" in your life? Here are five tactics you can try. Not sure where to start in decorating your apartment? Here are five ideas. Desperate to go on a date with the hot new guy in PR? Go with these five tried-and-true strategies.

So live that fabulous life you've always longed for: ditch the unnecessary responsibilities that are holding you back, let go of your inhibitions by trying something new, or dare to tackle that challenge you never thought possible. *The Essential Five* will help you dip your freshly pedicured toes into any unlikely endeavor!

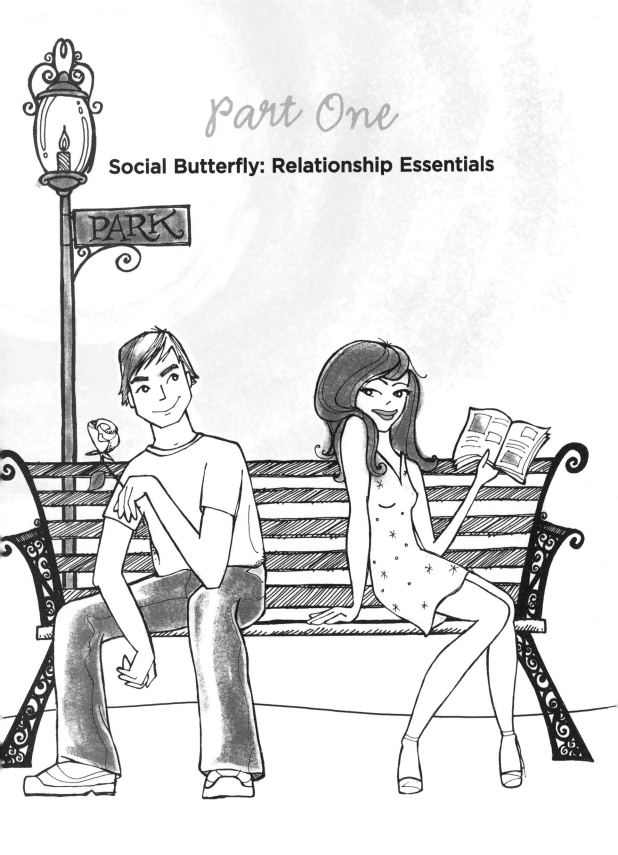

Part One

Social Butterfly: Relationship Essentials

Questions to Ask
on a First Date (and Some You Shouldn't)

First date jitters. It's that same nervous feeling you had prepping for final exams—*If I screw this up, my life is over. I have no chance ever again at finding true love. I will die an old maid surrounded by dozens of cats.* However, we all know that's not really the case, don't we? Look at the first date as an interview—and *you're* the one doing the hiring. Does he inspire you, enhance you, entertain you, thrill you? Here are some good topics to get started.

Are you married? While you may not want to phrase it exactly that way, it's crucial to find out about his background. Is he on the rebound? Is his best friend a total jerk? Is he devoutly something other than you are, or does he belong to a group you're opposed to? Does he have a criminal record? Some of these details can be nailed down by googling him; some will need to be asked (in subtle ways, of course). You can start the conversation in a nonthreatening way by volunteering info about yourself to get him talking: *When my ex-husband and my dad, who's currently incarcerated, by the way, once came to pick me up from protesting with PETA . . .*

Come here often? Everyone likes to laugh—everyone *needs* to laugh, in fact. Sven Svebak, a Norwegian researcher, has shown that having a sense of humor can prolong your life![1] So show him your funny side. Use a cheesy pickup line if that's your style. Tell a story about something goofy that happened to you. Or if you prefer, tell a straight-out joke. You'll either end up laughing hysterically or bored to tears. And really, either one is a good result—you'll know if you're meshing or not.

How much money do you make? Imagine being that forward on a first date! And wouldn't it be nice info to have? But while you can't ask him to hand over his most recent pay stub, you can find out if you have similar financial dreams and goals for your life. Are you expecting to live the high life—Upper East Side loft, Chloe Bay Bag-of-the-Month Club, society parties, and charity balls? Maybe he's dreaming of the simple life, with a small franchise to run in the suburbs, soccer practice on Saturday mornings, and a quiet night out at Applebee's as a special treat every once in a while. Find out what circle he runs in and if you want that to be your circle too.

If the idea of a first date terrifies you, consider hiring a dating coach! Patti Feinstein is America's Dating Coach, and if you visit her Web site at **www.pattifeinstein.com** and book her services using the promo code "FIVE," she'll give you a 10 percent discount!

What makes you tick? Most people really like to talk about themselves, and you show you care when you ask about their interests. So ask him about his pet peeves. What was the most fun he had this week? What was frustrating to him? When did he feel a sense of accomplishment? Don't interrogate, but you can find out a lot about his work life, his extracurricular activities, and his personal style of living when you get the conversation headed in this direction.

Check out this rash. Equally important to asking the right questions is avoiding the wrong conversation topics. Do not mention your ailing aunt, your most recent skin condition, your missing kitten, or—under any circumstance—your ex-boyfriends. Focus on the positive instead of the curiously depressing. Even if it's a good, heart-wrenching story, save it for later. You're here to shine, and turning into Debbie Downer is no way to brighten his impression of you.

Ways to Reconnect with
Your BFF, Your Archnemesis, or the Cute Guy You Had a Crush on in Algebra

With all respect to Deng, it can be hard to reconnect the lines of communication when years have blurred them. You have changed a lot in the last however-many years, and you're sure your friends have too. So how do you find your friends in the first place, and then what do you do once you've made contact?

Biggest slacker. If you don't love the idea of spending hours online or on the phone tracking down everyone you used to know, track down that one old friend whose strength and passion is just that. Once you have her onboard, your workload will be much less.

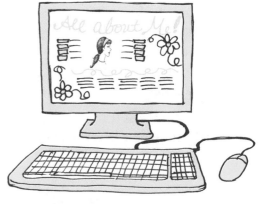

Most likely to succeed. Reuniting is made much easier with the Internet in our lives. (How in the world did people plan high school reunions twenty years ago?) Sign up at a Web site designed specifically for connecting old friends, or grab your yearbook and search for your friends on MySpace or Facebook. (Unbelievably, MySpace has more than 70 million members, dominating the Internet networking world.[2] Surely you can find a few people there!)

Wittiest. You don't have to wait every ten years to have a reunion, nor do you have to go through the effort it requires to gather people from across the country, never mind the world. Throw a spontaneous party for an old group of friends who live nearby! Let the invite spread through word of mouth, and gear up for a night of flashback memories, embarrassing moments, and hilarious stories you've never heard before from the "glory days."

Most artistic. The route involving the most work, but which could give you the most personal satisfaction, is to create a Web site with current news and pictures of your life. Add a contact page where people can e-mail you. Then the next time an old friend thinks of you and decides to google you, he'll come across your Web site and be able to get in touch! Add a blog with basic day-to-day details (only those you don't mind the whole world knowing about!) so people can see what you've been up to, and add funny bits in there to spice it up: "Won an Academy Award today. Fun. Think I'll put it in the bathroom."

Best all-around. A meaningful idea for a reunion is to meet somewhere that was significant to the group. If you all attended the same school or university, meet there. Or if you worked together, meet at what was your favorite lunch hangout. Make the reunion a real-life trip down memory lane.

Those truly linked don't need correspondence. When they meet again after many years apart, their friendship is as true as ever.

—Deng Ming-Dao

Secret Strategies for a

at Relationship with Your Mom

"What do you think, Mom?" Is your mom the overbearing, overprotective, drive-you-crazy-with-her-constant-phone-calls type of mother? She wants to do everything for you, because she knows you can't do it as well as she can. At least that's what you think she thinks. Well, indulge her every once in a while. Ask her opinion, and then take it. Buy something she thinks is cute. Let her tell you how to organize your pantry. Go out with the guy she thinks is perfect for you—who knows, maybe mother does know best!

> *My mother had a great deal of trouble with me,*
> *but I think she enjoyed it.*
>
> —Mark Twain

"It's on me." Everyone knows you're a proud, self-sufficient adult who does not need Mommy to pick up the tab for lunch, your dry cleaning, *anything*. But sometimes Mom just wants to believe you're still her little girl. And part of that is paying for stuff for you. So don't be so quick to be Miss Independent all the time. Occasionally let Mom pay for your special day out or even just for your run-of-the-mill errands.

a grown-up girl's handbook for everything

"I've got all day." How many times do you talk to your mom on the phone and find yourself anxiously glancing at the clock—or multitasking while you catch up? If you're living in a state of constant "I'm gonna be late to do something else]" in your relationship with your mom, it's time to slow down. Clear your schedule. And waste some time. If the two of you are chatting about how nice a manicure and pedicure would be, jump in the car and go get one. If you're visiting her for the weekend, turn your BlackBerry off. Be lazy with her—accomplish nothing. It may just be the best time you spend!

"Let's get outta here." Are you and your mom best friends? You like to imagine yourselves as Gwyneth and Blythe or Kate and Goldie—hip, young, adventuresome, but most of all, close. So spoil your mom by hitting the road with her—schedule a trip for just the two of you. A relaxing long weekend at the spa, a high-class shopping spree to your favorite big city, or a kitschy summer camp for adults where you can experience late-night bunk-bed chats, horseback riding, and canoe trips! Or let someone else do the planning: you can go to **GutsyWomenTravel.com** to join a travel program designed for women, and if you enter "GWTFIVE" in the promotional code box at checkout, you'll get $100 savings on your trip!

Be rude. Now, your mom would not approve, would she? Be rude to her? Huh? Well, when your mom comes to visit, she doesn't want to feel like any other guest in your house. She wants to feel special, like she's an insider. So don't play the perfect hostess when she comes over. Let her do the dishes if she wants. Don't wait on her hand and foot—just let her feel at home. She'll feel like a real mom again, and you might even get some help with the chores!

"I've become my father. I've been trying so hard not to become my mother, I didn't see this coming."

— Jennifer Anniston as Rachel Green, *Friends*™ © Warner Bros. Entertainment Inc.

7

Questions You Could Ask
a Complete Stranger

You know the drill. You're on the subway, in the crowded café, at the packed lecture hall. Everyone sits staring blankly ahead, reading the paper or listening to an iPod. No one talks. If you're tempted to break some social mores and strike up a conversation with that cute guy, interesting woman, or somehow-familiar fellow passenger, here are some tips for how to get the conversation started.

End-of-workday questions. If you're headed home from work and it's pretty clear your fellow travelers are too, generic comments like "Whew! Sure was a Monday, wasn't it?" or "Glad the day is over?" are fairly unthreatening, albeit pretty lame. In an effort not to completely bore the person you're talking to, and to show them you are, in fact, an interesting person, be on the lookout for something that connects you to them. Maybe they're sporting a logo for a brand based out of your hometown. Or ask if they like whatever new high-tech gadget they're fooling with. You may learn some helpful tips or even develop a new relationship for your business network!

Succumb to curiosity! Be bold and you'll be surprised. Whether you're dying to know what hair stylist she uses, where she bought her stroller, whether he is happy with his expensive parka (the one you were thinking of getting for your boyfriend), don't be too afraid to ask. You have a legitimate question, and people generally love to talk about themselves or something they have recently done or purchased. It gives them an opportunity to rave or complain to someone who wants to listen.

Ask for an opinion. Sometimes the people in your life are just too close to an issue to give you proper perspective, and you don't feel like shelling out big bucks to go see a shrink or other expert for advice. So ask a stranger! People generally enjoy sharing their opinions. You don't need to go into too much detail, and you should probably ask if they mind before you start sharing the full story. But you could end up getting a really unique viewpoint by asking someone who knows nothing about you. It could even be the best advice you get!

Pay it forward. Don't let curiosity, boredom, or loneliness be your only motivation to start a conversation with a stranger. Instead, communal transport can be the perfect place for an act of kindness, which will probably be a lot more fulfilling than a random conversation. So hand the sick woman a cough drop or a fresh bottle of water, pay the fare for the guy who's searching frantically for his wallet, or stop to pick up papers for the teacher whose bag has torn in the middle of the crowd. You can even join the Pay It Forward Movement at www.payitforwardmovement.org.

Don't speak to strangers! Perhaps the reason talking to strangers doesn't come naturally to us is because we were always told by our parents, "Never talk to strangers!" Old habits die hard. So, is there any truth to that old adage now that we're adults? Of course! Here are rules to safeguard you when talking to strangers: Rely on your intuition and don't talk (or continue talking) to someone who gives you a "bad" feeling. Never divulge any personal details. Be shrewd when it comes to handing out business cards. You can have interesting conversations with strangers while maintaining your anonymity.

New Family Traditions
You Should Start This Year!

Family day. There are national holidays for different members of your family—Mother's Day, Father's Day, and even the lesser-celebrated Grandparents' Day. So why not set a date every year to celebrate your *family*. Have a personal and intimate celebration with your immediate family or a huge blowout with your entire extended clan—crazy aunts, uncles, and cousins included. The more the merrier, right?

> *There is no such thing as "fun for the whole family."*
>
> —Jerry Seinfeld

Family historian. Every family should have its own historian. If the idea appeals to someone, let him or her run with it. Each family member will have his or her own interest in the family history and unique ideas about how to add that information to the family's growing historic records. You can report your favorite findings at your annual Family Day!

Volunteer together. Giving doesn't come as naturally as getting, but it is an incredibly rewarding habit. Take the initiative and choose a charity for which you and your loved one, or your whole family, can volunteer together. Ring bells for the Salvation Army or wrap gifts at United Way. Check out VolunteerMatch.org to find an organization that fits you.

> *Happiness is having a large, loving, caring, close-knit family in another city.*
> —George Burns

Create your own holiday traditions. Whether it be a "progressive dinner" (where you have a different course at each friend or family member's home) at Thanksgiving, a family Easter egg decorating day, or a cookie-baking evening before Christmas, creating your own holiday traditions will make these events more about your time together and less about the commercialism we all so easily get caught up in.

Urban family. More and more people today live away from home and get together with family only once or twice a year. If you're one of them, don't throw aside family traditions or spend the holidays moping about missing your family. Gather your urban family (your friends, neighbors, and all those who feel like family) around you and celebrate together. Create fun and unique traditions with this group just as you would with your own family.

Questions You May Not

Want to Ask—but Need to—Before You Say, "I Do."

Is he rich? All kidding aside, have you two talked finances? Are you on the same page with your expectations for the future? Do you treat yourself to Prada and Jimmy Choo with some regularity? Does he ration his toilet paper to save on spending? If you are coming from different sides of the financial tracks, make sure you're on the same page before you join your hearts and bank accounts in holy matrimony.

Does he complete me? Channeling Jerry Maguire and his ultracheesy romantic side may not be your guy's forte, but it's important to ask yourself if you're looking to him to make yourself whole. Are you emotionally healthy enough to be in a relationship this serious? Are you sucking the energy, inspiration, and motivation out of the relationship, or are you adding those things to it? Would you want to marry you?

It takes a mighty good husband to be better than none.

— Mary Engelbreit

Do we have chemistry? While your guy may be smokin' hot right now, he's still gonna look less like Brad Pitt and more like Frank Costanza over time. So, even though your physical chemistry is important, step back from that for a minute and take a good look at your friendship. Is it going to get you through the romantic dry spells? Is there more to your relationship than fireworks?

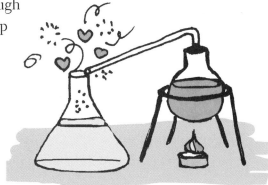

Does my mom like him? You've heard it before—when you marry a guy you marry his family. The thing is, it's true. If your family has strong reservations, or if his does, you should seriously consider them. You need to come up with a battle strategy for winning over their affections, and the first step is to stay on the same side. When faced with a choice between defending your guy and defending your mom, you may be emotionally distraught. But if you guys are married, you'll need to be on the same side, have each other's backs, and make your home a safe place where you can feel protected.

Do I respect him (and, does he respect me)? Your beau may be cute, funny, wealthy, and Harvard-educated, but do you respect him? It's a major question you need to face before you take the plunge. Why? Because even in this twenty-first-century world where women are strong and men are metrosexual, it's still important for your guy to be a stand-up man you don't mind deferring to. Now your most pressing issues are which restaurant to eat at and which movie to see, but down the road it will be how to discipline your kids and whether to move to another city for his job. If you don't truly respect each other's opinions and decision-making abilities, you'll be very unhappy. It's time to fess up—is each of you willing to put your dreams, your hopes, your life into the other's hands?

Battle Strategies
for Taking On Nosy People

Some people just have to know everything about everyone all the time. Here are some strategies for maintaining your privacy with even the peskiest of busybodies.

Overinvolved parents. Boredom, anxiousness, a different idea of personal boundaries—there must be a reason why your mother-in-law feels she can tidy your underwear drawers while she is house-sitting your home! She probably misses the time when she had kids at home to take care of and longs for those days again. Give her some small area of responsibility and make it a huge honor to ask her. Or tell her some news, and make a big deal about your telling her first. Letting her know that you're keeping her involved and in the loop might be all it takes.

The blabbermouth friend. Do you have a friend who spreads all your news for you? She's the expert on your life, and you kind of feel as if you've become her personal reality show. Although you could take it as a compliment she finds you so interesting, no one likes to be gossiped about. So how do you politely end this debacle? Exercise great caution in giving her big news first— and make sure you've told anyone you want to tell personally. But don't cut her off completely; it will send her imagination flying, and you never know what theories she might come up with—and share with everyone!

Your boss. All e-mails sent from your work account can be read by your employer. "What?" you ask. Yes. Anything you send across your company's server can be stored there, and your boss has a legal right to read it. So get a separate account for your personal messages and be really strict about keeping business, business.

Strangers on the Internet. Identity theft, one of the fastest-growing crimes in America today, involves criminals obtaining your personal information, usually to buy things on credit or empty out your bank accounts. So, to avoid having this happen to you, make sure you never give out your Social Security number, whether online or elsewhere; use a good antivirus program; always use a "secure" server when transmitting credit card information over the Web; and never give out unique personal details unless you know whom you're talking to.

Your kids. Children have a way of getting you into the stickiest situations. Whether they've repeated something you've said, called you out in public, or walked in on you in private, you probably realize some boundaries need to be drawn. Rig an alarm for a toddler's bedroom door so you have a few precious seconds to grab some clothes when the alarm goes off! Be sure—double and triple check—you are alone before you have an incriminating conversation about a personal situation or vendetta! And, finally, have a sense of humor. You're going to be embarrassed by something they say at some point, so try to just laugh it off and move on.

Things to Say or Do When
a Homeless Person Asks You for Money

How do you first react when a person with little sense of personal space accosts you on the street? All he wants is some cash, but your defenses go up immediately. What is the right thing to do? And how do you know when to help and when to bolt?

Look him in the eye. The eyes are the window to the soul, or so the old adage goes. You can tell a lot by looking in someone's eyes, whether you know the person or not. So take a good look. It will influence your generosity and will also play a role in your personal safety. People are much less likely to attack someone who looks them in the eye with confidence.

Give her something. If you decide this is a person you want to help, you have lots of options as to what you want to give her. Cash, of course, is always one way to go. But if you feel uncomfortable with that, other options are gift cards to fast food restaurants or, for the brave of heart, actually inviting the person to eat a meal with you! You could also give clothes, toys, books, or bottled water—keep some in your car for just that purpose.

16

Teach him to fish. The old Chinese proverb says, "Give a man a fish, he will eat for a day. Teach a man to fish, he will eat for a lifetime." So how does this apply? Maybe you know someone who works for a cleaning services company that hires unskilled workers for the night shift. Get a bunch of her business cards to keep on hand, and give them to people who "will work for food."

Run away. It is a noble thing to help others, but you have to be aware of what's going on around you. If you're downtown at night, in the dark, alone, you're not being smart. Carry mace or pepper spray, and be ready to run. Do a quick mental check of your self-defense moves (see "Things You Need to Know to Defend Yourself from an Attacker" on pages 208-9), and protect yourself. Don't try to be a hero when your chances of coming out on top are low.

Let it sink in. The situation this person has found himself in is not one he dreamed of as a little boy. Chances are, small things went wrong too often, until big things went wrong and he found himself on the streets. Be grateful for what you have. And if you want to know more about the plight of the homeless from a personal perspective, pick up the book *Same Kind of Different as Me* by Ron Hall and Denver Moore.

Possible Reactions to
Encountering Bratty Kids in Public

You're out for a nice dinner after a long day at work, and the kid at the table next to you starts hollering and throwing his food. You decide you can't take it anymore when his open-faced peanut butter sandwich hits you smack on the forehead. Here are your options:

Denial. Probably the most commonly accepted response to witnessing naughty children in public is to just ignore them. They're not your kids; it's not your problem. You can breathe a sigh of relief that you're not the one having to go home with those little devils. Chalk it up to another good dose of birth control—you are *so* not interested in having kids right now!

Make a mental note. When you see a five-year-old running the wrong way up the escalator, climbing over the edge, and jumping off to land on her little brother, you look around for the responsible adult watching these ruffians. All the women nearby, however, are oblivious to the situation. Who is the mother here? Why is she not taking care of this? At this point you make a mental note: I will *never* let my child act this way in public. Keep a journal back home of all the "nevers" you promise yourself. They'll be good reminders—and probably make for a good laugh or two—when you do have kids of your own.

The beady eye. So, you've figured out which mom is allowing her precious little princess to run around the bookstore screaming bloody murder while she uses her oh-so-cute Lelli Kelly sequin-encrusted boot as a weapon on any unsuspecting bystander. Your next level of involvement is the prolonged glance at the mom. By staring deep into her worn-out soul, you're letting her know you see this behavior and it is "unacceptable." You are her personal Supernanny, and it is time for the naughty corner.

Say something. Oh, for goodness' sake, not to the parent. Your next option is to say something to the person you're with . . . so that the "responsible" adult in the situation can hear. Here are some options: "Oh my. That little boy looks as if he might get hurt banging his daddy's *steak knife* against the table *over and over and over again.*" or "You know, when I was at the dry cleaner's *this morning* picking up this *expensive cashmere wrap*, he warned me that I should be very careful to make sure I don't get anything sticky on it—like *jelly*, for example."

Be the jerk who actually gets involved. There are a few situations in which it's appropriate to actually step in and say or do something when kids are behaving badly. Of course, if you have a child who is in danger in any way— about to get smacked in the face with a hammer or pushed off a slide on the playground—you can kindly correct the offending party and save your child from imminent harm. Or, if the kids are being so annoying that it's actually ruining your evening, say something, but be nice. Give the parent an out, like: "I'm sure you didn't notice your child is whacking my head with her princess wand, but would you mind asking her to keep her spells to her dolls?" or "I'm having a bit of a hard time hearing the movie, and I'm sure you are as well. Do you think it might help to go walk the baby around?" The most important thing to remember if you do decide to go this route is that you shouldn't feel guilty about saying something—that will only ruin your night further.

Ways to Heal
a Broken Heart

Cry. When you're feeling rejected and abandoned and really angry, it's important to have a good cry. In fact, scientists have discovered that crying releases the negative hormones in your body, thus keeping depression at bay.[3] So stock up on the tissues, and let it out! Grab a pillow or a punching bag and hit something. Don't be afraid to be a mess for a day or two—if you've been wronged, and it's totally normal for you to just get it all out.

Ice cream. It's time to spoil yourself. Take a day or two and do whatever you want. Take the day off from work (your heart *is* broken, remember!), watch sappy movies in your pj's, and eat all the ice cream you can stomach.

Breaking up is hard to do.
—Neil Sedaka and H. Greenfield

Delete his phone number. Sweetie, it's sad but true: it's over. You cannot be his friend right now. It's just too confusing. It's time to pack up the mementos, delete his number from your cell phone, and pretend like he doesn't exist for a while. Eventually you may be able to rekindle a nice platonic friendship, but you need some *time*. So get over him by forgetting him . . . for now.

Journal. Just like a good cry, writing your emotions down Bridget Jones–style can be cathartic. Don't censor yourself—you can always burn that journal later! Write it all down, every pang of distrust, every name you want to call him, every twinge of "if only," every last little iota of hope—get it all out on paper. It helps to speak your mind, even if you're the only one who hears.

Take charge. This is a new day and a new era in you-ness! It's time to take on the world. Ignore that negative self-talk trying to beat you down. You can do anything! Find a new project and devote yourself to it wholeheartedly. And go for more of the find-a-new-outfit, get-a-new-haircut, save-dying-kids-in-Africa type project, not the new-hottie-in-Apartment-3G type.

Ways to Answer
Annoying Questions—and How to Ask Some of Them!

In a 2007 presidential debate a college student went to the microphone and asked John McCain a tacky question about his age. McCain was faced with the classic dilemma of how to answer a really rude and annoying question. He humorously responded the way many of us wish we could, "Thanks for the question, you little jerk. You're drafted."[4] Here are some scenarios you might face:

How much do you weigh? There is no reason for anyone to need to know this most personal of numbers unless you're a contestant on *The Biggest Loser*. But if someone dares ask such a tactless question, you can respond by simply saying, "Gosh, I'm not sure, I don't have a scale on me." How to find out: Other than spying, there's really no good way to find out, and no good reason to.

How old are you? Some women are ashamed of their age—whether it's their youth or their maturity they're trying to hide. While you should be proud of who you are at every stage of life, it's fine to avoid revealing your birthday if you don't feel in the mood. Laugh them off and say, "Twenty-nine, again!" How to find out: Beat around the bush—"What did you wear to your prom?" or "Where were you when the Challenger exploded?"—to put the pieces together.

How much do you make? How to respond: "Oh, we do fine," is a perfectly acceptable response, or use some humor: say "one million dollars" in your best Austin Powers imitation. That is, if you aren't standing there dumbfounded that someone would ask such a personal question without any tact. How to find out: Research comparable salaries in the field your target works in to get a range of salary potential.

Have you had plastic surgery? How to respond: If you have had surgery and don't want to admit to it, just deflect the question and respond to the "compliment" instead. "Oh, you're so sweet! No one's ever asked me that before!" If you haven't, own your amazing assets—"No way, I've worked hard for this body!" How to find out: Look at old pictures and compare.

Why did you go to the doctor? How to respond: Let's face it—many times our trips to the doctor are not something we want to broadcast in the office newsletter. You can come up with a false condition to avoid the question with humor—"Oh, just to find out about this highly contagious rash I've got," as you take hold of the asker's arm. How to find out: Express your concern for her without going into details—"I hope everything's okay. Let me know if I can help in any way."

Things You'll Never
Understand About Men . . . So Why Even Try?

They can't (or won't) multitask. We women are used to driving the car while we put on makeup and chat with our best friend about our current work dilemma. Men don't work this way. They do one thing at a time and focus on it completely. You'll find yourself calling, "Honey!" five or six times before he turns his attention away from the game. Science has proven that men can't multitask like women can, and many men have wholeheartedly embraced these findings! So embrace it too—when he's entranced in his phone call, that's the perfect time for you to sneak in and put away those new Christian Louboutins.

They get over it . . . fast. Men don't hold grudges the way women do. They fight and get over it—end of discussion. So let's learn a lesson from our male counterparts. If your girlfriend has offended you in some way, work it out and leave it in the past. Don't relive the hurt or embarrassment in your head (or through phone calls or in e-mails) for days and weeks to come. You'll feel much lighter when you're not carrying around resentment.

Just because they say it, doesn't mean it's so. Guys like to think out loud. They'll throw ideas around to get feedback, but it doesn't necessarily mean they're going to do it. For instance, "Honey, I'm thinking about going back to get my master's in archaeology this fall." Now, if you had said that, you'd have thought it over for weeks before coming up with the perfect way to broach the subject, the exact phrasing to get him to agree with your decision.

So he wants to go back to school! Wow, you'll spend exotic summers on digs in faraway places, seeking fame and fortune. How Indiana Jones of you! But next week he grunts a confused "Huh?" when you ask if he's sent in any applications. Alas, that idea has passed. This week he's aiming for a spot on the PGA tour.

Where's the . . .? Guys tend to lose things. Why is it that a man can have lived in a house for years, yet still not know where you keep the bath towels or the broom or the spatulas? Is it possible that he doesn't *want* to remember? So when it's time to put away the laundry or clean the floors or empty the dishwasher, he's utterly helpless. It always seems easier to just do it yourself. Hmm . . . interesting.

What he sees in you. You've got your boss breathing down your neck, your mom is always on your back, and the bank is tightening its grip on your finances. So you're a little hard on yourself—you notice all the negatives and tend to ignore the great stuff. But your guy loves you—he thinks you're great, flaws and all. Embrace that—don't waste your time wondering what he sees in you or convincing yourself that he can't be that interested. If all you show him is neediness, then that's all he'll be able to see.

"Men and women belong to different species, and communication between them is a science still in its infancy."[5]

—Bill Cosby

Ways to Let
Your Parents Know How Much They Mean to You

Mother knows best. Mom never stops being "Mom," no matter how old either of you gets. She has advice for you every step of the way, and because she is always ahead of you in life, she probably knows a thing or two more than you do. As familiar as your mom is, and even though you realize more and more about her natural human shortcomings as the years go on, don't overlook her when you need advice, an opinion, or a shoulder to cry on. And don't ignore her if she gives it to you without your asking.

Don't hold your parents up to contempt. After all, you are their [daughter], and it is just possible you may take after them.

—Evelyn Waugh

Time well spent. Livingto100.com says, "People who do not belong to cohesive families have fewer coping resources and increased levels of social and psychological stress . . . associated with heart disease, various cancers and increased mortality risk."[6] Yikes—who knew avoiding your parents could cause cancer? Well, it's not that simple, but you should do what you can to build a

a grown-up girl's handbook for everything

meaningful, even spontaneous relationship with your parents. So plan a vacation with them—even if it's just for a couple of days. Send them a scrapbook or video of highlights from the year. Write them a note to let them know what you appreciate about their character. Do what you can to keep the family close.

Be a decent person. "I have no greater joy than to hear that my children walk in truth."[7] This sums it up for most parents—they want to sleep soundly at night not worrying about what their kids are up to, what trouble they might be in this time around, or who might be influencing them the wrong way. Living in such a way that makes your parents proud is a great way to honor them. They can brag on you to all their friends, be confident that you're contributing positively to society, but most of all, have a clear conscience that they raised a good human being.

Give your parents a helping hand. I know it might feel like the minute you walk into your parents' home they whip out a to-do list that they need your help with. But instead of feeling used and abused, see it as a way to help your parents maintain a good lifestyle—after all, they did change a lot of dirty diapers and wipe a lot of runny noses for you! Plus, if you know they're comfortable, you won't have to worry about them as much.

"Never underestimate a parent's ability to mortify his child."

—from *The OC*™
© Warner Bros. Entertainment Inc.

Celebrate them. Your parents' twenty-fifth wedding anniversary or sixtieth birthdays only come around once, so there's no better time to give back and really show them what they mean to you. Invite all their friends and family and throw a memorable bash in their honor. These are the few occasions you can even get away with a soppy, heartfelt "what you mean to me" speech.

Ways to Make
a Man Fall in Love with You
(for the First Time or the Millionth)

You've spotted him—tall, dark, and handsome; confident, blond, and athletic; short, nerdy, and bespectacled. Whatever it is that floats your boat, he's got it. And you're crazy about him! So how do you go about making him crazy about you? Here are some tried-and-true ideas.

Just be yourself. It's okay to act nervous, be the initiator, or tell dumb jokes. If he doesn't like *you*, you're wasting your time anyway. And if you can tell he's inwardly rolling his eyes at you, remember that some guy will find your story captivating, your quirky smile stunning, or your goofy joke hilarious. Hold out for him—he's the one you want anyway.

Flirt a little. A guy wants to feel as if you find him attractive—that's not just a girl thing. So flatter him. Be affectionate. Even be willing to be a little . . . creative. Liven up a relationship gone flat with some tender loving care. Treat yourself to some silky, sexy lotion or some fabulous lip plumper from Avenue You's online beauty warehouse. (And if you use the promo code "FIVE" at their **www.aveyou.com** Web site, you'll get a 15 percent discount!) Slip into something comfortable, and treat your hubby like he's the king of the castle.

Ignore him. Hard-to-get is a game of subtle nuances and thin lines between right and oh-so-very-wrong. It's not being his ultimate fantasy one day and an ice queen the next. It's not turning a blind eye to his advances. It's letting him know that you are a real prize, not just any old girl he can conquer. If he wins you over, he's really accomplished something—because you are a great catch!

Love his mom. There is a special bond between mother and son, and you can maximize your impact by subtly taking control of this relationship. Now, I'm not suggesting you act like Kate Hudson in *How to Lose a Guy in 10 Days* and make her a scrapbook with photos of what your kids will look like, but if you make an effort to genuinely like your crush's mom, it will win you points with him and with her. The key is in letting *him* know how much you enjoy her, not telling *her* everything about your relationship.

Don't embarrass him. Did he say something really lame at dinner the other night that the two of you laughed over for the rest of the evening? That's great that he has a sense of humor about himself. However, don't mistake it as an invitation to blab his faux pas to all his friends. They may laugh, but he won't appreciate it, and, ultimately, they won't either. Instead, look for opportunities to make your beau feel superconfident about himself and his relationship with you when he's with his buddies. When he realizes you have his back, that's a significant moment in your relationship.

Romantic Ideas
for a Valentine's Day You Won't Forget
—and Neither Will He!

Romantics. For couples who are unashamed romantics, and staunch traditionalists, an evening beginning with red roses and champagne while watching the sunset, followed by a candlelit dinner and then by nibbling on chocolate during a romantic movie is perfect! Or you could even watch the sunset from the vantage of a hot-air balloon ride by calling **1-800-SOARING**, which has two hundred locations nationwide, and using the promotional code "FIVE" to get a $30 discount.

Gift-givers. Flowers. Candy. Lingerie. Jewelry. Fancy dinners. If your heart speaks this language of love, splash out and make this year memorable! The later you start on your gift-buying quest, however, the more difficult it becomes. Keep an "ideas" list throughout the year, and when you know you've come up with the perfect one, don't be afraid to go ahead and get it early. Planning ahead could save you money that you could use to buy some additional last-minute gifts, which will only make the day even more special.

Romance is the glamour which turns the dust of everyday life into a golden haze.

—Amanda Cross

Jet-setters. If you and your hottie share a passion for traveling, what could be better for the annual celebration of your love than a trip to a romantic destination—a favorite spot or one you have never visited before. The weather in Maui is good year round. Nothing beats the excitement of New York City. And the food is great in Florence. So check on your frequent-flyer miles and book yourself a special surprise getaway!

Adventurers. For the outdoor couple who loves action and adventure, nothing is more romantic than getting that natural adrenaline high . . . together. Never been skydiving before? Ready to tackle that hiking or canoeing trail you've been eyeing? Get online and search for some vacation packages that cater to your wild side. Give your Valentine's Day an edge by taking a daring trip together!

I love romance. I'm a sucker for it.
I love it so much. It's pathetic.
—Drew Barrymore

Nonromantics. If the thought of getting all gussied up to go out for a way-too-expensive dinner makes you nauseated, or if you think getting a huge bouquet of flowers at work is just something to make your coworkers jealous rather than a beautiful expression of sincere affection, romance may not be high on your list of wants. So, what do you do on this high holy day of passion and love? You and your sweetie pie can bond over a romance protest! Beer and burgers for dinner, a great action flick, and lots of laughing at all the couples working so hard to be so deep, so sincere, so over-the-top. You get the picture. You'll celebrate your love for each other much more this way than you would with any candy heart box or pink balloons!

Ways to Make Sure
You Don't Ruin a First Date

"You never have a second chance to make a first impression." How many times have you heard that in your life? First dates can be stressful—I mean, this could be the guy you'll spend the rest of your life with! This could be your *last* first date ever! Are you crumbling under the pressure? So how do you calm your nerves in this torrent of anxiety?

Be *fashionably* late. If he's coming to pick you up, don't make him wait more than five minutes. If you're meeting him out somewhere, same deal. You'll probably need to try on ten different outfits before you find the one that perfectly conveys your personality in a single glance, but making him wait speaks volumes more than Marc Jacobs ever could. Pull out all your tricks—set your clock ahead, write the time in your date book thirty minutes early—to make sure you are prompt.

Don't try to impress. The only thing more obvious than a person trying too hard is hanging a big sign around your neck that says, Like Me. Love Me. Marry Me! And if you're going out of your way to impress someone, you're probably not really being yourself. It's easy to look at a first date as a test you have to pass, but in reality you're checking to see if this guy is suitable for *you*! So forget the total-body makeover, the

32

borrowed clothes, the impressive vocabulary, and the sudden interest in everything fantasy football—just be yourself. There's no point in forcing a fit.

Play hard to get. Don't get physical on the first date. Leave him wanting more!

Thank him afterward. If you're interested in the guy, let him know you appreciated his asking you out. Send him an e-mail, or even better, a handwritten note telling him you had a great time. He'll see that you're courteous and considerate—definitely good qualities that guys want in a girlfriend. But beware of coming across as needy: don't sound as if it's the first date you've had in months (even if it is) or as if you're dying for him to call you tonight (even if you are).

Have an escape plan. Sometimes you know—and soon—that it's just not going to work out. In that case, have an exit strategy. You can simply tell him honestly but tactfully that you appreciate his generosity in taking you out for a nice dinner-movie-football game, but that it just might be time to call it a night. If you're more of a people-pleaser, have a friend call you an hour after your date starts. She can be your excuse to get out of there fast. But remember that this guy, even if he isn't for you, may very well have some cute friends, and you don't want them hearing bad things about you. So be kind when you let the loser down.

Friends You Really Need
to Have in Your Life

Some people have tons of friends. Others have only a few very close friends. You may feel obligated to be friends with certain people. You may wish you were friends with others. And many of us know at least one friend we'd rather not have. Here are five types of friends you need in your life.

The mentor. Find someone twice your age, or at least ten years older than you, who you can go to when life gets tough—someone who will listen to your crises and give you advice about all your major decisions. She will be honored that you want her wisdom, and you can only benefit from verbalizing what you are going through. Getting the perspective of someone who's been around the block once or twice before is really invaluable.

The trusted friend. Whether it's honest but loving advice regarding how your backside looks in a pair of pants, or a truthful opinion about something personal, having a trusted friend is a must. They're are hard to come by and it takes time to identify them, but once you've found a friend you can trust, you have usually found a friend for life.

The banter buddy. You're a chatterbox who would make any *Gilmore Girls* fan proud, and you need a gossip outlet. So who's the Rory to your Lorelai? You know that you can't call just any friend and talk for hours—only certain people share your same gift. Embrace the woman who considers endless hours of chatting one of life's great luxuries. But before you start racking up the cell phone bills, put her in your network or set a date during off-peak hours to call.

The play pal. You have to get out of the apartment, do what you love, let off some steam, but it's never as much fun without a friend. Who do you know who's always up for something spontaneous and is willing to make the time? You've found your play pal. Whether it's tackling a DIY home improvement project, taking a cooking course, or joining a community softball league, your play pal will make it all the more fun with her infectious energy and laughter.

The protégé. Have a look around you: is there someone half your age, or at least ten years younger, who could do with an older "sister" in her life? You can start out by keeping an eye and ear out for what she needs and calling her up for an occasional lunch date. Soon your protégé will become as much a friend to you as you are to her, keeping you younger and surprising you with her insight into life.

Ways to Win
a Fight

Avoidance. In some cases, but not all, the best way to win an argument is to avoid it altogether. This mainly applies to confrontations with people who will argue about anything—they seem to thrive off the drama. It's as if these people have an evil superpower that enables them to absorb your energy and leave you drained. Resist the urge to bite back when they confront you. Remember, that's exactly what they want you to do.

Choose your battle. Your in-laws are mad that you won't sign up for their Republican Party fund-raiser. Your sister is peeved that you prefer the blue plates to the orange ones for your mom's birthday party. The key to choosing your battles is in making sure you truly believe in the issue up for debate. It is equally important to know you can win the argument and that the payoff is really worth the fight.

Don't become the adversary. You never want the person you disagree with to regard you as an adversary. If she starts out on the defensive, it will be much harder for you to persuade her. Avoid using the word *you* if you can. Rather than saying, "You're wrong," say, "My opinion is . . .," while making it clear that it diverges from hers. And do your best to make her say yes. By agreeing with you on little things, you're introducing her to the idea that you two *can* agree.

Let them lose. An argument can sometimes be won by letting your opponent talk. People love to talk and they love to hear themselves talk, so listen carefully, because your opponent's explanation may give you the information you need to win the argument.

Admit your mistakes. Make an effort to appreciate that people have different opinions, and try to see the situation from your opponent's point of view. If you realize you are wrong, admit it immediately. Don't be tempted to become like those people who can never be wrong and forgo logic and facts in a desperate attempt to "win" the argument. Being humble enough to admit fault is an admirable quality, that people will respect.[8]

"When people work together, there is going to be conflict. You can't outrun your problems. And that is why the idea of a cage match is so universally appealing."

—Steve Carrell as Michael Scott, *The Office*

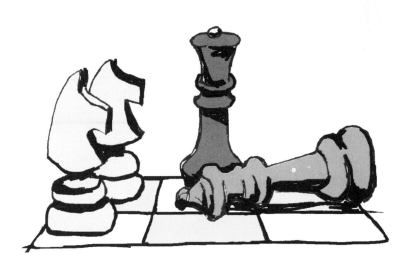

Ways to Let Them Know
How You Feel

Every woman has her own unique love language to express how she feels about others. And we all have a way in which we prefer to be shown we are loved. So what's your language? The love languages descriptions below come from *The Five Love Languages* by Gary Chapman.[9]

Do something. When someone you know needs something, do you immediately think of ways to help him or her? He's starting a new business—hey, you know a lawyer who can help out! She recently had a baby—and you organized a schedule so they'd have meals brought to them for two weeks straight! You're a doer, and it means so much to you when someone takes the time to help you when you need it. If this is your style, you don't need any extra motivation from us! Just knock yourself out making a difference for your friends. But be careful not to overdo it—you don't want to wear yourself out *or* come across as a know-it-all.

Time. It's one of those roll-your-eyes adages that you've heard a million times, but it's true: "love" is spelled t-i-m-e. It applies to almost any relationship—with kids, parents, friends, lovers. But when someone goes beyond simply spending time with you and makes a sacrifice to do it—he skips poker night with the guys to go to the opera with you or gives up his spot in the raid on his video game to help you get the kids bathed and put to bed—it really makes an impact. If time with you is what he wants, be willing to make a sacrifice every now and then; you'll be glad you did.

Gifts. It's very genteel, very formal . . . almost quaint, isn't it? The gentleman suitor arrives, gift in hand, to win the heart of his fair maiden. It's the stuff of Valentine's and romance novels. If this is how your guy communicates, embrace it and recognize it as his way of expressing his love. And if he likes to be loved this way, take a moment to think of something he'd really like to have and surprise him with it.

Touch. You know your husband loves you most when you're making love. You feel your mom's love for you most in her warm, sturdy hugs. And you show your best friend you love her when you're there to hold her hand as she gets the results from the doctor. This is a great way to communicate your love for others, because it's free, it's always available, and it's easy to give away . . . for you. Keep an eye out for those who are uncomfortable with physical intimacy though—not everyone appreciates a kissy-kissy greeting or a playful pinch on the bum.

Tell them. It's obvious, isn't it? But sometimes you just need to hear those words: *I love you*. Your need to be appreciated, understood, and respected is universal. So use your language to strengthen, motivate, and lighten the load for those you love. And be compassionate toward those who truly struggle to get those words out. Don't withhold your love just because they have a hard time verbalizing theirs—look for other ways they may be telling you their feelings.

Fun Christmas Gift Ideas
for Those People You Hate to Shop For

***Away* in a manger.** For those family members who have everything and are just plain impossible to buy for—like Mom and Dad, the in-laws, or even your significant other—the gift of a weekend away to somewhere they wouldn't usually think to go, couldn't afford to go, or wouldn't normally take the time to go is sure to be the best gift they will receive this year. And if they'd like it, go along with them! There's nothing like a vacation to create memories and bring family closer together.

The man with all the toys. With a little research, you can easily find out what the latest gadgets are, and with minimal fuss you will not only have a unique gift but a Christmas conversation starter. But beware: these gifts can create envy in those family members who don't receive the "latest" whatchamacallit this Christmas. Look for innovative toys for a niece or nephew, electronics gadgets for your dad or brother-in-law, or a nifty kitchen tool for your mom or sister.

Think of giving not as a duty but as a privilege.

—John D. Rockefeller

God *rest* ye merry gentlemen. Who works like crazy for your family—always offering to help when needed, cook a meal, watch the kids, organize the parties—but rarely gets any thanks in return? The gift of pampering might be right up her alley. A certificate for a back massage or a manicure and pedicure may be just what she needs, especially after the busy holiday season. If your hubby is the one you want to treat, consider some personal pampering: perhaps a handmade gift certificate for a candlelit bubble bath with champagne and sushi for two.

I'll be home for Christmas. If you can't make it to be with your family during the holidays, send pictures! We all love to have photographs of our loved ones around the house, but finding the time to organize all your prints and get them framed or put together a photo album is not easy. Pick your favorite photo from the year—one that captures a memorable time together—and have it framed. Or go online and create a photo album with old treasured photos and scanned-in handwritten family recipe cards, fun and silly pictures from the family reunion, or just a "year in the life" of your family for them to share. Log on to **picaboo.com/ideacenter** for some great ideas, and start yours today! If you enter "1P25PO-FIVE" in the promotional code box at checkout, you'll get a 25 percent discount!

Joy to the world. If the overcommercialization of Christmas bothers you, make donations to charities on behalf of your adult family members this year. (The children may not understand your disillusionment with gift giving at Christmas, so you may want to leave them out of this one!) Spend the time you would have been traipsing the aisles, trying to come up with the right presents, doing a little research on charities to make sure the ones you choose are legitimate and that your money will actually go to those who need it. World Vision makes things easy for you with their charity catalog—you can buy a goat for a farmer, provide educational support for a child, or give hope and assistance to a sexually exploited girl. Log on at www.worldvision.org.

Ways to Dump 5
Your No-Good, Very-Bad Boyfriend

It's over. You've seen it coming, but now it's here, and you know it's time to end it. You have to ditch your guy. But how? Your method of getting the message across may depend on the length, type, or intensity of relationship you shared. Be kind. Be clear. And be concise.

Text message. Americans rated this the worst possible way to break up with your significant other, but with our modes of communication becoming more and more relaxed, love-struck romantics are getting blindsided by their cell phones every day. Breaking it off via text message is *only* okay if there's not really a relationship there to start with. Maybe he thinks it's more than it is. Maybe you've been on one date and you're not really interested in saying yes to the weekend in Aspen he just invited you to. Note: keep this most casual of communication methods for the most casual of relationships.

Write a letter. Getting all your grievances, all your thoughts, all your dashed dreams and broken hopes out on paper is a good way to speak your piece without interruption. You can think through your message clearly, and you can edit yourself—make sure you don't say something you'll regret later. If you're a bit intimidated by the prospect of ending things, and you're a little unsure of yourself when you're speaking off the cuff, you might want to consider spilling your guts on paper. Note: if this is a serious relationship you're talking about here, you'll be the better gal if you hand it over in person and make yourself available to talk things over after he's read through it all.

The fade. Although not the gutsiest of approaches, many people have successfully pulled the fade on their significant others with few repercussions other than confusion and bewilderment. You simply turn down his requests for dates . . . gradually becoming more and more distant. He'll eventually get the picture that you're not interested, and he'll start asking other people out. It's the nonbreakup breakup. Note: this is best reserved for guys you've only been out with a few times.

Talk it out. For the brave, confident, go-getter girlfriends . . . or maybe just the really, really mad ones, a heart-to-heart conversation is the way to go. Let him know you're just not feeling it anymore. He's done something specific that's hurt you, and you will not be able to get over it. Or maybe it's you— you're wanting different things from life than he's offering, and you're not willing to give those up for this relationship. Note: Having this conversation takes a lot of guts and a lot of honesty. Prepare yourself for the emotional and mental battle that lies ahead.

Set him up. No, not for failure. Set him up on a blind date. If you're truly over this guy, you're sure you will never want to date him again, and you have no fear of burning bridges, then this can be a fun way to break it off. Find someone who's willing to be your blind date girl, and give her your message. (This can be a friend of yours—a coconspirator, if you will; or it can be a random acquaintance who might actually fancy going out with the guy.) She'll communicate your feelings for you when he shows up for what he thinks is dinner with you. Note: this approach is best reserved for cheaters and other low-down, dirty, lying jerks.

Ways to Keep
the Romance Hot

You may be dreamily in love or struggling to figure out if this guy is the one for you. Or maybe you're already committed but searching for some of that spark that seems to have gotten lost amid the piles of laundry and dirty dishes. You feel that most of the advice you read is really far-fetched and totally not *you*. Here are some simple ways to keep the fires burning without changing who you are to get there.

Keep quiet. Believe it or not, even the cherished words "I love you" can become mundane and meaningless over time if used too often or flippantly. This phrase can too easily be used as a cop-out to make amends for strain or distance in a relationship, instead of being a passionate expression of the true emotion. So find other ways to let him know the same thing: be specific about why you love him. And sometimes even saying, "I like you," can have a lot more significance than "I love you."

Speak his language. The old saying "Actions speak louder than words" has endured the test of time because it is so very true. If you don't already know, take the time to learn what says "I love you" most to your partner (read "Ways to Let Them Know How You Feel" on pages 38–9). Next time you're tempted to throw a quick kiss or "I love you" his way, take a moment to give him a shoulder massage, ask him how his day has been, or offer him something to eat or drink.

Spoil yourself. You love to shop, right? So why not take a little time during your lunch break to buy something you know *he'll* really enjoy. Stop by your favorite lingerie store for a no-special-occasion surprise for your hubby. You'll feel extra sexy in something new and spicy, and he'll love watching you model your purchase.

Ditch him. Everybody needs time alone. Granted, some people need more time alone than others, and since opposites usually attract, most likely one person in your relationship will need more space than the other. If you're the extrovert, don't take this as a personal insult. Your guy just needs more space and time than you do to get peace of mind. When he's feeling overwhelmed, organize a girl's night out to give him some privacy. Or if he's the extrovert, encourage him to do the same with his guy friends.

Get away together. Your work schedule has been so crazy that you suddenly realize you've only spent about two hours of quality time with your man in the last two weeks. Or, when you convinced your mother-in-law to take the kids for the night, you ended up sticking around the house, catching up on laundry and other chores. It's high time for you two to get out of the house and have a romantic getaway—whatever that means to you. Rent a cabin in the woods, visit New York City—even if going to a movie and eating out once a month is all you can manage, make sure you do at least that.

Things You Need to Say
to Your Boss

Whether your boss is a megalomaniac like Montgomery Burns of *The Simpsons*, a complete imbecile like Michael Scott on *The Office*, or a ruthless fashionista like Miranda Priestly from *The Devil Wears Prada*, you have to deal with your boss every day, and she determines much of your day-to-day happiness—not to mention your salary, vacation time, and chances for promotion. So what can you say to her to make sure she's got your back?

"I thought you should know . . ." Keeping your boss informed about your work progress, as well as significant happenings around the water cooler, will ensure you stay in his inner circle. Don't tell him about every e-mail you send, but do let him know where you're having successes and where you're having trouble getting things done. And only communicate the essential bits of gossip to him—you don't want him to think you're a tattletale, but he will appreciate knowing that his employees are grumbling about the slow response his customers are getting from accounts payable.

"I know what I'm talking about." When you propose a new client, a change to the way current business is done, or a creative way to cut costs in your business, know your stuff. Your boss won't take you seriously if she doesn't think you've done your homework, prepared your pitch well, and considered the suggestion from all angles. Wow her with your smarts—this is the time to be a know-it-all!

"How can I help?" If you see your boss is overloaded with work from his superior, or if he has to make up some slack your coworkers have left for him, step in to help. Offer to prepare the PowerPoint for your department's presentation to corporate, ask if you can pick up lunch for him when you go out, or remind him that it's his secretary's birthday next week. Eliminating the little stuff from his to-do list will help him realize what a valuable member of his team you are—and he'll remember that when it's time for your performance review and raise!

"Actually, I think you're wrong." If you're in a team brainstorming meeting, a small strategy and development session, or a one-on-one status update meeting with your boss, don't be afraid to express your contradictory opinion on the subject at hand. She'll be impressed by your gumption and confidence in your beliefs, and she'll appreciate hearing another side of the issue. But beware of saying this to close-minded, arrogant bosses; they'll likely respond negatively to direct opposition, so choose your words carefully!

Nothing. Know when to sit along the sidelines and let your boss do the talking. If you're going along for a pitch to a big potential client, don't upstage your boss. If he miscommunicates an inconsequential detail, just write a note to slide his way—don't correct him in front of the board of directors. And if the gang is bashing him at lunch, don't join in. You never know who could be sitting nearby who might take the details of the conversation—and your lack of involvement in it—back to him.

Ways to Find a Boyfriend
for Your Best Friend

Your friend has been single long enough—it's time to get her a guy. But she's unwilling to do the blind date thing, is snobby about the Internet, and is too shy to ask out any of her guy friends. What's a girl to do? Take things into your own hands. It's time for an intervention. Here are some ideas to save the day.

Post it. Put her profile on a dating Web site on the sly. Use a fantastic picture. Write a glowing review. And pay for her subscription! Now all you have to do is wait for the calls to come in, which you're sure they will by the hundreds!

Host it. Do you know the guy who's just perfect for your gal pal, but she's been unsure about doing the blind date thing with him? Make her comfortable by hosting a party and inviting them both. Make it a casual cocktail party where neither of them will feel threatened or set up. Just make a simple introduction with good details— "Jill is part of a Pulitzer-winners book club, and Jack here just published his first piece in *The Atlantic* last month." Let them progress in their own time.

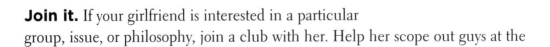

Join it. If your girlfriend is interested in a particular group, issue, or philosophy, join a club with her. Help her scope out guys at the

PETA meetings, the Young Republicans mixers, or the church's singles events. You can be her wingman as she voyages uncharted territory.

Break it. Your plumber is so darn cute, and you think he'd be great for your friend. Loosen her pipe fittings, then give her his number. Or maybe she is terrible at her finances and your accountant is a real gem—make an introduction and get her an appointment with him. Subtly let your set-up guy know she's available, then arrange a nonthreatening businesslike meeting. If he asks her out at the end, all the better!

Leave it. It is possible to push too hard, which only turns a girl away from the idea of dating even more. So when you have her primed and ready, back off. Let her go forward at her own pace. Don't repeatedly call and ask how it went. Don't beg her to get back in touch with him if she's not ready yet. The last thing you want is for either of them to resent your involvement.

Part Two

Classy and Fabulous: Lifestyle Essentials

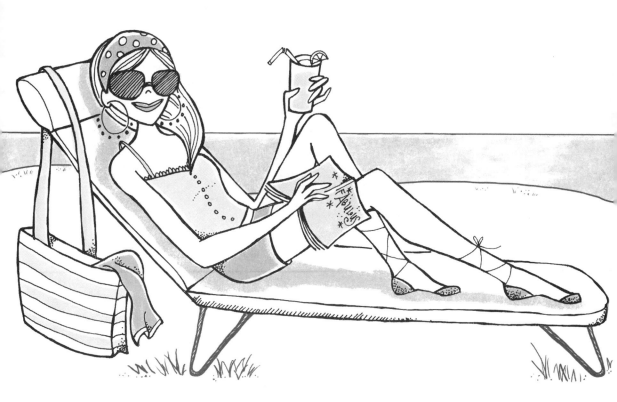

Strategies for Surviving
Awkward Business Functions

You're at a convention out of town and have to attend an awkward networking event disguised as a "party." Or it might be a company-wide event to celebrate your latest financial goals. Either way, you have to be on your toes at an office party—making introductions, meeting new people, and being charismatic. Yippee. So how do you survive a social event with those you would probably never choose to socialize with?

Greet the host first. This isn't just good manners but the quickest, easiest, and smartest way to meet people and begin conversations at a company function. The host invariably knows the most people in the room, and it is her job to make sure everyone is having a good time. So make your presence known! Give her your name, a quick compliment (on her home, the invitations, whatever), and a bit of info about yourself that she can pass on when she introduces you to someone nearby (which she'll automatically do if she's a good host). And away you go! You will no longer be an awkward wallflower.

Make a bold introduction. Charging up to your boss's boss or the exec at another company you'd love to work for is not worth the effort unless you make a bold introduction. Be confident and impressive as you greet these fellow partygoers. But do your homework before you go: find out who will be attending, decide on two or three people you would most like to meet, and then put your best foot forward. With a drink in hand and a radiant smile, introduce yourself, deliver a handshake without spilling hors d'oeuvres on your dress, and do your best to carry on a stimulating conversation. Hint: the best way to hold someone's attention is to ask questions about him or her.

Stay in the safety zone. The Massachusetts Institute of Technology's Sloan School of Business, which offers a crash course on cocktail party basics, counsels students to loiter by the food table rather than the bar. That's because people tend to grab their drinks and move away from the bar, but they are more likely to linger near the food. Not only that—people's endorphin levels are higher when they're close to food, which boosts their memory and the chance that they'll remember you later.

Flatter someone. Always come to a company function armed with at least three conversation starters about your work, your industry, or news related to your business. If you can't come up with any, you can seldom go wrong with flattery, as long as you make it sincere. As Michael Scott, the boss on *The Office* television series, so eloquently puts it, "I don't want somebody sucking up to me because they think I am going to help their career. I want them sucking up to me because they genuinely love me."

Talk about current affairs. Never resort to the mundane, dead-end, "How are you?" type of questions. Catch up on the latest current affairs so, if all else fails, you can ask people what they think about the issues going on in the world at the moment—whether it's the latest castoff from *American Idol* or the exit strategy for the war in Iraq. And if they haven't done their homework or aren't familiar with the topic themselves, you can fill them in (and look pretty smart in the process).

Carey McBeth-Cooper, founder of Vancouver-based Essential Etiquette, says that when people are representing their organizations at business social functions outside the office, they should keep in mind that "you never know who is going to be at that function, or who is watching you, so certainly your behavior in that situation is critical."[1]

Prayers
to Inspire Your Soul

A Prayer of Protection. Circle me, Lord. Keep protection near and danger afar. Circle me, Lord. Keep hope within. Keep doubt without. Circle me, Lord. Keep light near and darkness afar. Circle me, Lord. Keep peace within. Keep evil out.[2]

A Prayer of Love. Lord, you are my lover, my longing, my flowing stream, my sun, and I am your reflection.[3]

A Prayer of Perspective. All shall be well, and all shall be well, and all manner of things shall be well.[4]

An authentic life is the most personal form of worship. Everyday life has become my prayer.

—Sarah Ban Breathnach

The Lord's Prayer. Our Father in heaven, hallowed be your name. Your kingdom come. Your will be done, on earth as it is in heaven. Give us this day our daily bread. And forgive us our debts, as we also have forgiven our debtors. And do not bring us to the time of trial, but rescue us from the evil one.[5]

The Prayer of a Mother. Dear God, I thank You for the gift of this child to raise, this life to share, this mind to help mold, this body to nurture, and this spirit to enrich. Let me never betray this child's trust, dampen this child's hope, or discourage this child's dreams. Help me, dear God, to help this precious child become all You mean him to be. Let Your grace and love fall on him like gentle breezes and give him inner strength and peace and patience for the journey ahead. Amen.[6]

Ways to Keep
a Modicum of Privacy While Working in a Cubicle

DWIGHT: Please knock, this is an office.

JIM: (pointing to a sign) It says *workspace*.

DWIGHT: Same thing.

JIM: If it's the same thing, then why'd you write *workspace?*

—from *The Office*

Monitor your monitor. You probably don't have a say in where your cubicle is located or of the desk layout inside it, but you can arrange your belongings to suit your privacy needs. Step number one should always be to choose the most discreet spot for your computer. Place your monitor so that it will get the least amount of over-the-shoulder exposure to prying eyes—you may not want your neighbor to know that you're complaining about her stinky perfume or your boss to know that you're surfing for shoes online during your break.

Create boundaries. The biggest problem with cube privacy is that there isn't a door, and for that reason most coworkers feel they have a right to walk into your cube whenever they want. Friendly-looking BUSY or DEADLINE signs set up at the "door" to your cube, or even hanging from a rope barring the entrance, is an easy solution to this problem. But beware: office door etiquette is a sensitive topic. Fending off the coworkers too often or for too long can earn you a rep as unsocial, "not-a-team-player," or even rude.

Repel cubicle lurkers. Every office has its busybodies who get twitchy when things are too quiet for too long. These social butterflies are sure to pop into your cubicle at random times during the day when they need some conversation and company. At first you may be flattered that they want to talk to you, but when your deadline is fifteen minutes away and you're getting the gory details on Alice in Accounting's latest foul-up, it can be a real nuisance. Two tips for keeping cube lurkers away: avoid eye contact as they pass by and put something in your guest chair or any other "seat" they could possibly fill.[7]

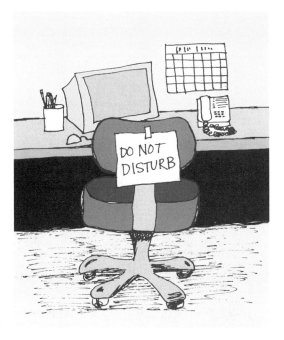

Don't forget Big Brother. Someone in your office—usually the systems administrator—is watching all of the e-mails that come and go from your computer. So, although you may be tempted to forward the latest bawdy joke or e-mail a piece of gossip about a fellow workmate, resist the urge! According to experts, if your e-mail system is owned by your employer, the company is legally allowed to review its contents.[8]

Surviving extreme setups. The "joys" of sharing an office cubicle are not unlike those you experienced back in junior high when you had to share showers in the locker room after soccer practice. Just as it was back then, it is important now to define your separate spaces. Split things evenly, and check in regularly. Ask your cubicle mate to tell you when he needs quiet or more space. This will give you the right to politely request the same from him when you need it.

Childlike Qualities
You Should Never Lose

We all wish we could be kids again—to be able to enjoy the bliss of having someone to cook and clean for us, take care of us, and most important . . . to have lots of time to play! Girls just want to have fun, right? The truth is there are some fun childhood practices we could benefit from bringing back into our lives.

Play outdoors. While we don't *necessarily* need to run around playing cowboys and Indians in the backyard with the neighbors, we need to make time to be outside. Remember how often you played outdoors as a child, riding your bike around the neighborhood and running around in the park? Mom had to make a rule for you to come back inside by nightfall or in time for dinner. How has your life changed? How much time do you spend stuck inside a cubicle or behind a sales counter? Find creative ways to get outside. If you have the flexibility to do so, take your work out of the office. If not, plan some outside activities for the weekend—whether it's a hiking trip, drinks on the patio at your favorite hot spot, or a relaxing afternoon by the pool.

Find delight in the small things. Go up to any child and tell her she is about to get an ice cream cone, and then capture the look on her face: pure excitement! As life's challenges become bigger and our aims become higher, we must remember to be thankful for everything we have, even the small things. So relish a rainy Saturday morning when you can snuggle under the covers a bit longer; enjoy a long line at the grocery store as it gives you a chance to catch up on pop-culture gossip, or try to remember every moment of a good hug or a good cry.

Create. Childhood is all about being creative—making up games and stories, playing dress-up, drawing and coloring pictures . . . the list continues. How much time do you give yourself to dream, to be creative, and to carry out your ideas? How often do you get the satisfaction of having created something yourself? You don't have to paint a picture to hang above the mantel, but there is a great sense of satisfaction and achievement in decorating your home, decorating a cake, or planting flowers in the bed in front of your house.

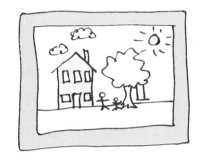

Admire someone. As a child, you looked up to certain adults with unabashed adoration, to women you wanted to be like when you grew older. You modeled yourself after them and came to them with puzzling questions. But as we grow older, busier, and more cynical, the list of people we look up to and who actually have an influence in our lives grows smaller—often disappearing altogether—as we try to convince ourselves and others that we have it all together and don't need help from anyone else. So start looking up to someone you admire and can learn from, and keep your eye open for someone younger than you whose life you can enrich as well.

Throw a tantrum. Your boss is being a major jerk. Your bills are overdue. Your mom called *again* to find out when you're going to get engaged. And the dog is sick. Sometimes you need to let off a little steam, and it's okay to channel that inner three-year-old and throw a good old-fashioned tantrum. Not that you need any ideas, but here are some that come to mind: Scream! Just belt it out at the top of your lungs. Have a good cry. Go to a kickboxing class and hit something. Spend money. Just get it out so you can get over it and move on.

Spas Worth Traveling Around
the World For

Every girl enjoys the lap of luxury every once in a while, and what better way to pamper yourself than with a day at the spa? These are the Crystal Award–winning spas of 2006—the crème de la crème of the world's spas, according to SpaFinder.com. So pack your bags—there's one winner for each continent that has a spa. (Someday we'll be traveling to Antarctica for mud baths, but not yet!)

Africa's Santé Winelands Wellness Centre. Do you love being in the mountains, eating world-renowned organic food, and living in ultimate privacy? Then this is the perfect spa for you. Get ready for first-class services and specialization in restorative privacy and a quiet retreat. The spa's signature offering is *vinotherapy*: massage, scrubs, and hydrotherapy utilizing grape seeds, grape-seed oil, and the extract of red grape skins.

Asia's Chiva-Som. Are you inspired by exotic settings, royal tradition, and holistic treatments? This stunning retreat boasts fifty-seven individual pavilions in traditional Asian architecture overlooking the Gulf of Thailand. It is the summer residence of the royal family of Thailand, and guests to this spa are treated like royalty as well. The spa features adventurous cuisine and high-tech treatments for ultramodern connoisseurs.

Australia's Spa Chakra Hayman. If your idea of relaxation and opulence requires a beachfront location, then you can do no better in the Great Barrier Reef. Built around stunning lagoons and peaceful waterfalls, this private island getaway offers penthouse suites or private villas with views of the spa's lush gardens or the Coral Sea. With exclusive access to Guerlain therapies, a patented facial and body massage technique developed in Paris in 1938, this spot has a unique attraction to spa connoisseurs.

Europe's Brenner's Park Hotel and Spa. If city living is more your style, you'll love mingling with upper-class Europeans at this spa in historic Baden-Baden, Germany. The classic décor of this 130-year-old institution is quite grand, but some rooms also offer the minimalist furnishings you'd expect to find in Sweden. The full beauty and medical offerings are eclectic and exciting—from the peaceful Japanese blossom steam bath to the unique "torture massage" for the adventurous. Guests laud the "impeccable and discreet service" provided by Brenner's staff.

North America's Miraval. If you need some time away from your hectic life, too much stress, or even a chance to escape from a recent tragedy in your life in a relaxing and restorative environment, Miraval is the perfect destination for you. This spa focuses on bringing life into balance by practicing "mindfulness," so you may attend a program where you learn to balance a feather in your hand or develop self-knowledge through grooming horses.

South America's Kurotel Longevity Center and Spa. If you're looking for a spa experience that will challenge your senses, inspire your spirit, and heal your body, Brazil's Kurotel, located in the heart of a dense forest, may be just the place for you. The founders of the spa envisioned a center with the "sophisticated resources of a hospital, the capabilities of a beauty clinic and fitness center, and the comfort of a hotel."

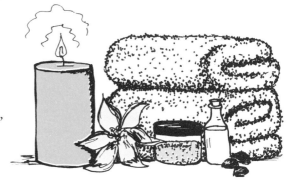

Tips for Tipping a Waiter
So He Won't Spit in Your Food!

Health magazine ranked being a waiter as one of the ten most stressful jobs you can have.[9] No wonder—with complaining customers, fussy kids, ornery cooks, and a similar to an obstacle course work environment—these men and women really do "work hard for the money"! So, how do you keep your waiter on your good side?

The basics. We all know you should leave at least 15 percent of your total as a tip for the waitress in the US. Most of these servers rely on tips for a large percent of their income. So don't stiff them. Don't claim bad math skills as an excuse either—it's not that hard. If the service was decent, add $1.50 for every $10.00 you spend. If it was good, add $2 for every $10, or even more. And Suzanne, a waitress in Tennessee, told us if you accidentally leave the "customer copy" of the credit card receipt on the table and take the "merchant copy" home with you, the waiter gets gypped out of his or her entire tip! So pay attention.

Eating with the kids. Even though you may have children, it doesn't mean you are never allowed to leave your kitchen for meals. And you don't have to relegate yourself to nice lunches out at Wendy's as your special treat. It's important to teach your children good restaurant manners, but while they're still in the learning phase . . . be kind to your waiters. If she's going to have to do a deep carpet clean, or if her other customers are looking a bit unhappy that they've had to listen to "no, no, no" during their entire lunch, do what you can to make up for it in an extra-nice tip.

The long, leisurely lunch. It's so nice to go sit at a restaurant with a close friend and linger, talking over anything and everything that comes to mind. Before you realize it, you've been at it for three hours, and the waitress is glaring at you from behind the hostess station. He could have turned that table over four times—and gotten four times the tip he'll get from you. So, if you're out for a gab fest, let the waiter and hostess know beforehand that you're planning to take awhile—that way the waiter will be prepared for your stay, and the hostess might seat a few extra groups in his area to make up for your slow lunch. But be sure to leave a more generous tip than normal to make up for his losses.

Where everybody knows your name. Do you have a favorite restaurant? The waiters know your name, you have a "usual" order, and it just feels like home when you're there? Your generosity will spread through the staff there, and they'll fight over getting to serve you. If you have a regular waitress, get her something a little extra at Christmas or for her birthday—a gift card for a massage or manicure. You'll get top-notch service in return: "Didn't care for the soup? Let me get you something different. Want another glass of that yummy fruit tea? Here's one in a to-go cup so you can take it home with you. You just got engaged? Dessert's on us today!"
Make them love you there, and
you'll enjoy the service even more
than you already do.

There goes her tip! Sometimes you encounter the rudest of rude waiters. The ones who seem to have forgotten we exist. The ones who spill things on you or bump the back of your head with their tray, without as much as a halfhearted "sorry." When the service is truly terrible—the waitress was offensive or genuinely incompetent—and you're sure it's her fault, not the kitchen or the management or the general environment in the restaurant, your refusal to tip can be a message to the waitress that this is perhaps not the field of work she should be in.

Things to Do When Everyone

Is Telling You, "You Need to Get a Life!"

Does your typical day go something like this: wake up, go to work, come home, pop dinner in the microwave, and spend the rest of the evening vegging out on the couch? Or maybe you're chasing after kids all day long and you have no energy left at the end of the day to even wash your hair, much less get dressed up and go out! Here are some easy things you can do to add some spice to your schedule!

Check the papers. Look through the Living or Weekend sections of your local paper for fun (and often free!) local events going on. A festival at the park, jazz night at the art museum, or the Little League championship game downtown are all surefire ways to break your dinner-and-a-movie rut. Grab some friends or go with your honey and hit one of these hot spots for some good conversation and lasting memories. The movies will always be there for you later on DVD!

Host a party. Whether it's an open house for your whole address book or just an intimate dinner with a few friends, get some folks together for a good night of fun! Play cards or parlor games, crank up the music for an impromptu dance, or play a game of backyard baseball. Or, if you and your friends all have kids, rotate having a party for the kids one night a month so that the other couples in your circle can have a life for a few hours!

Quit something. You're more than likely overbooked, overscheduled, and overworked. You're so busy doing stuff that you have no time to do things you want. So quit something—pick one of your responsibilities and drop it. Instead, do something for yourself—take up painting, practice yoga, or read a book. Your new knowledge will give you great conversation topics, and you'll feel more satisfied with yourself.

Get active. Quit spending your evenings on the couch and go take a walk. Go to the park for a picnic dinner and feed the ducks at the pond. Go for a hike or bike ride. Walk to the neighborhood café with your boyfriend for dinner. You'll find that when you get moving, you'll also get talking.

Give back. Charity work is a great way to meet people, fill up your calendar, and feel really satisfied with your time. Philanthropic work can range from serving meals at a homeless shelter to attending formal balls with thousand-dollar dinners. You can find a way to help others that fits your schedule, your budget, and your interests. Ask around at your place of worship, look online, or talk to friends to find an opportunity that fits your personality and lifestyle.

Things You Need to Know
About Your Money

Ginita Wall, a nationally recognized expert on the subject of women and money, offers the following truths about women and money in her book *It's More Than Money—It's Your Life*, coauthored with Candace Bahr:

A man is not a financial plan. Whether you are married, single, or somewhere in between, you can't depend on Prince Charming. You are likely to be handling money on your own during part of your adult life. So what's a damsel to do? Taking responsibility is the key. If you are married, you need the skills to be able to stand on your own—especially since we women tend to live longer, earn less, and save less for retirement. Each month, after the bills are paid, figure out where you stand financially and discuss your plans for the following month with your partner if you have one. Failing to discuss financial issues can jeopardize your security individually and as a couple. Disagreements are inevitable, but you should be able to discuss your differences openly and settle them fairly.

You can't succeed unless you start. Procrastination is a common obstacle, especially for women. Men may put off taking important actions out of sheer laziness or complacency. For women, procrastination usually stems from fear. Many women avoid taking control of their finances because they're afraid of failing—and disappointing their family. Others are afraid of succeeding financially because of the responsibility money entails. But overcoming these fears is critical to ensuring your financial security. If you are afraid to face your financial future, you'll blindly spend your money instead of saving it. Get started now, and you can create financial security for yourself and your family.

Think small for big success. The journey of a thousand miles begins with one small step, according to the Chinese proverb. The same is true of finances—the best way to begin is, well, to take a small step forward. Sometimes we think that we have to make major changes to get back on track. But in reality, major changes are the result of a series of small steps. As you learn to think small, your confidence in your ability to handle your finances will grow. So start a savings account. Increase the contribution you make to your 401(k). Cancel any credit cards you don't need. The little things will add up over time!

Saving a little can mean a lot. The less you have, the more savvy you need to be when handling money. Many women feel they don't even have enough to get by, so there's no point in creating a plan for their future. But a small salary shouldn't keep you from living the high life! Optimism and ingenuity are two key elements to making the most of your money. Saving a little can mean a lot over time. If you save just one dollar a day, that's $365 a year. It's not much, but it's more than you had before. If you save $5 a day for your entire working life, you could retire a millionaire!

Money talks. Money can't buy happiness, but it can definitely affect relationships. The last thing most women want to talk about when they fall in love is money, yet it's one of the most important things you can do. The two of you must be in sync about money issues, or else you'll find yourself fumbling forward into the future with few clear-cut goals and no plan for how to achieve them. To be a successful team, four attitudes are key: trust, shared goals, communication, and planning.

Ways to Avoid
Being a Lout on Your Cell Phone

Fifteen years ago my cell phone was "for emergency use only." Now every third grader on the playground has his or her own personal communications gadget, complete with Disney characters and GPS devices. And with the sudden surge in conversation that's swept the globe, our sense of propriety seems to have been lost. Here are the most annoying habits of cell phone users, and how to avoid being one of the worst of our kind.[10]

Do not wear your earpiece when you're not on the phone. Have you ever answered a question when you thought someone was talking to you but really she was on her microscopic earpiece? Your reaction upon realizing your blunder can range from flushed with embarrassment to hotly annoyed. But beyond frustrating in the ranks of annoying hidden-earpiece behavior is the overly important individual who keeps her earpiece on at all times, just in case anyone might want to talk with her at any given moment. Get over yourself!

Do not have an annoying ring tone. It's annoying enough to have to hear phones ringing during movies and meetings—but to hear "Sexxy Back" blare out at church or "Stayin' Alive" at a funeral is beyond unacceptable. Please pick a ring tone that is plain and simple—*ring ring*—and set at a low volume. Or better yet, keep it on vibrate when you're out in public.

Remember that you have a life apart from your cell phone. Your phone calls are important, and in this age of übercommunication, people expect you to be available at all times. However, please, please do not slam your BlackBerry or cell phone down on the table while you're enjoying a nice dinner with a friend. In essence, you're saying, "Someone more important might want to talk to me, and if that's the case, I want to be ready to ditch you as fast as I can." (As if you couldn't interrupt the conversation and leave her hanging if the phone was in your purse when it rang.) Take a moment to remember the days when you couldn't be reached 24-7. They were nice, weren't they? Set some cell-phone boundaries for yourself, and let voice mail pick up the message every now and then.

Don't yell. They can hear you. So can we.

Use your phone for good. There are many ways you can apply this rule to your cell-phone-centric life. For one, be safe. Use the voice-dialer feature on your phone when you're driving. Look where you're walking. Two, donate old phones to charity. Battered women's homes usually accept old cell phones for the women who come to them for refuge. And three, consider buying a phone that gives back, like the Product (RED) phones by Motorola.

> "Loutish cell use is out of control. Mobile phones now ring at weddings and funerals, job interviews and surgical procedures. No event is immune."[11]
>
> —Joanna L. Krotz

Tips for Taking
a Truly Memorable Vacation

Relax. What's that? When's the last time you did nothing? Skipped town, turned off your BlackBerry, and left all responsibilities behind? Unfortunately you might feel you aren't getting value for your hard-earned dollars if your vacation schedule isn't packed with activities every minute of every day. But instead of tramping through too many museums to remember, plan a day to sit by the pool and enjoy a good book, some great music on your iPod, and a refreshing piña colada. Relaxing is a truly novel concept today—something we all should do more often for our own health and well-being!

Vacation is what you take when you can't take what you've been taking any longer.

—Author Unknown

Make life interesting—do something unique. It's easy to get stuck in a vacation rut, going to the same destination or with the same people year after year. Granted it's familiar and safe—you know what to expect, and that's better than it being a disaster. Or is it? Maybe you need a little excitement in life—a complete change of scenery and lifestyle for a short while. Let your imagination run wild, and then go with it!

Plan well—but be spontaneous. The best vacations are well planned. Taking the time to investigate your upcoming trip and organizing an itinerary that suits your needs eliminates the stress of trying to decide what to do each morning or having to debate the next day's activities with the family each evening. You'll be more relaxed on your trip if as much preparation as possible is done before you leave. But if you have a Type A personality, watch out that you don't get bogged down by your plan. Keep your eyes and ears open for exciting or new opportunities. Throwing your schedule out on a whim can make the vacation that much more fun!

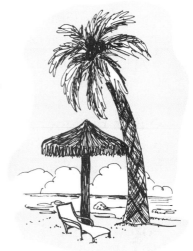

Pick an exotic destination, and go! Forget Disney World, Six Flags, or the family fun pack from your travel agent. Take the road less traveled and plan a one-of-a-kind getaway this year! If you're into the outdoors, Alaska offers hiking, kayaking, boat trips, and fishing. If you fancy the beach, visit Mazatlan, Cabo, or Cancun. Europe has an abundance of historic cities and beautiful parks! You could even plan a tropical vacation to Costa Rica's lush rain forests and rapids or a once-in-a-lifetime tour of America's top fields during the baseball season.

Pick the right travel companions. If it's a family vacation you're planning, then I suppose you can't choose to leave anyone "home alone." But before you jump in and make the compulsory invitations, consider the following: Will the family member insist on visiting every single historic building in a ten-mile radius when you're of the opinion that when "you've seen one, you've seen them all"? Is he or she a huge sports enthusiast while you'd much prefer to check out the shopping? In short, make sure your travel companion will complement your goals for the trip—not counteract them. You don't want to come home more stressed than when you left.

71

Ways to Pick a Book
You're Sure to Love

Don't you hate buying a book someone recommended, only to get halfway through it and realize that you absolutely hate it? And don't you love that feeling of discovery and hope that comes in turning each page of a really fantastic story? So how do you know how to pick a good book, and how do you avoid the losers? Here are some ideas to get you started.

Oldies but goodies. If a book has stood the test of time, if centuries after it was written it is still hailed as one of the greatest books of all time, there's probably something to it! So check out those classics. From *Moby Dick* to *Anne of Green Gables*, there's got to be something there that you'll enjoy.

Prizewinners. There are tons of awards given for books every year. From the Pulitzers and Nobels to the Caldecott and Newbery, from the Firecracker Alternative Book Award to the Gold Medallion Award for the best Christian book, there is bound to be an award that interests you. So go online and google your interests along with the words "book award." You'd be surprised to find there just might be a book award that fits along perfectly with your passion for Ben & Jerry's ice cream, hula hoops, or the GOP.

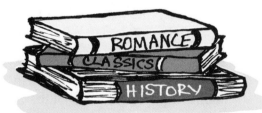

"Have you read . . .?" Probably the best way to pick a book is to find out what your friends have read and loved.

The reason this is so great is that you can ask in-depth questions before you take the plunge to actually spend time reading the book. Ask not only if *they* liked it, but if they really think *you'd* like it. Find out if they'd read anything else from that author. If you're not totally sure you're convinced, see if you can borrow their copy before you buy your own.

Be honest with yourself. If you're more of a *Bridget Jones* kind of girl, don't jump into *Atlas Shrugged*—try as you might, you're probably not going to love it. Read books that you will enjoy, rather than trying to impress anyone with your bookshelf. You're not in high school anymore—read what you want to read!

Don't buy the book. With mega–chain bookstores on every corner and Amazon serving your needs online, it's easy to forget we can get books for free in this world! So if you're looking for a good read, stop by your local library. Get the librarian to help you find something that suits your fancy. If you quickly discover you hate it, no sweat! You didn't shell out any hard-earned cash for it. It's a great way to do a "taste test" on a lot of books to see what you really love. Then, once you find some authors or genres that you realize you adore, you can spend your money building your personal library—and you can actually say you've read them all!

Just the knowledge that a good book is waiting at the end of a long day makes that day happier.
—Kathleen Norris

Web Secrets for When
You Want to Travel on the Cheap

You want to travel the world, but you're on a serious budget! Here are some secrets to travel in style without breaking the bank:

Travel deals. There are dozens of sites out there offering great deals for any type of globe-trotting jet-setter. These sites allow you to enter the specifics of your travel plans, and they give you the best deal around. It's like working with your own travel agent but on your own time.

Alternative accommodations. Did you see *The Holiday* with Cameron Diaz and Kate Winslet? In the movie they switched houses so they could vacation in other parts of the world. It's called a home exchange, and it's a great way to visit another city or country at minimal cost. Log on to **www.HomeExchange .com** and enter the code "FIVE" at checkout to receive a 25 percent discount on your membership! Another option for the more adventuresome traveler is youth hostels. There are hostels all over the world that allow you to bunk for the night for next to nothing. Check out more than ten thousand hostels at www.hostels.com.

Travel in style. You need great travel gear when you vacation, right? Picking unique luggage (or even just fun, flirty luggage tags) will help you identify your bags quicker at luggage claim, and you'll feel fresh and stylish at your exotic destination. So for trendy, hip luggage and travel accessories, visit www.TravelingChic.com. If you enter "FIVE" in the promo code box at checkout, you'll get a 15 percent discount on your purchase!

Live it up! While you're on vacation, the last thing you want to worry about is spending too much money in restaurants and bars, but you want to have a good time too! There's not much point in going to New York if you just eat McDonald's every day you're there. But eating out can be très expensive! Log on to www.valpak.com and enter the zip code for your travel destination. You'll be able to print out coupons for tons of great restaurants! Now you can dine out guilt free.

Stay home. Have you ever wondered what it would be like to be a tourist in your own hometown? Get some friends together and cheese it up! Do all the touristy stuff you can think of, eat out, and then head to someone's house for a slumber party afterward! It's like a mini vacation without the expense of traveling, and you'll get to see your city in from a whole new perspective. Visit your city's department of tourism Web site for ideas.

Surefire Tactics
for Getting a Great Flea Market Deal

The buyer's advantage. Sure, you really want that awesome antique side table you spotted across the stall, but you don't need to buy it as badly as this guy needs to sell it. So as the customer, you always have the upper hand. Hold out for the best deal possible; don't rush to say yes too quickly. Hint: Vendors don't want to pack their stuff up to take it home again—they want it sold! So you may get better deals the last day of the sale.[12]

Poker face. Stand in front of the mirror for a few minutes before you go, and practice your best "no deal" face. Don't appear overly eager to buy anything; instead, try to remain expressionless. The only time you should show emotion is to show disinterest in your seller's initial offers. Hesitation is a powerful tool.

Know your product. You'll feel a lot more confident negotiating if you know the retail price of the item you are negotiating for, but even if you don't, make sure you look it over thoroughly to find all its imperfections. Then use your gut to decide what you think it is worth. Know what you are willing to pay for it, and use its imperfections to leverage down the price.

Your first bid. You know how much you're willing to pay for something, but where do you start in your negotiations to get the best deal? A good rule of thumb is to take the max you are willing to spend and offer 40 or 50 percent of that. He'll come back with a number closer to the asking price, and you'll eventually work your way to some point in between.

When all else fails. If the seller's "final offer" is too high, your first recourse is simply to walk away. Often this spurs a desperate final attempt from the seller, which will likely be the lowest offer you will get. You can also hesitate and say you'll only accept that price if they throw in something additional.

Ways to Keep Your Perspective
When All Hell Breaks Loose

We all have those times when everything bad seems to happen at once—not only has the dishwasher leaked all over your kitchen floor, but your boyfriend is out of town for two weeks, your boss demanded that you finish a huge proposal by tomorrow, and you just spilled your Starbucks all over your newly detailed car and your brand-new cashmere sweater. You just want to scream. Here are some simple tasks for keeping your cool.

Have a mantra. Although you may feel like a lunatic doing it, you'll really calm down if you have a phrase you can repeat to yourself in the midst of the chaos. *This too shall pass. I deeply and completely accept myself. Serenity now.* Pick one and use it.

Take Baby steps. You can easily become overwhelmed when life packs in the punches, so fight back by picking one problem at a time and knocking it out. Make a list and cross things off—it provides a rush of satisfaction to rival any high.

Throw a tantrum. Go outside and scream—or stay inside and scream. Throw something. Hit something. Cry. Call an understanding friend and unload on her. Buy something outrageous—unless finances are on your list of problems! Do what you need to do to get it out, clear your head, and refocus so you can get back to a place of sanity.

Pick on somebody. That is, in your mind. Think of someone who's worse off than you and give an "Amen, hallelujah!" that you're not in his or her situation. Conjure up the image of your sister having to deal with her kids' incontinent gerbil, your coworker's meddling sister-in-law, or your archenemy's itchy skin malady. The funnier, the better.

Be a superhero. Psych yourself up for conquering the world. You can do it—you're strong, sexy, and smart, and you can take on the drama that's trying to take over your life. Stubborn, slow landlord—no problem for you! You'll call him every hour on the hour until he gets the job done. Sleazy, swindling car mechanic—bring it on! You're not afraid to get quotes from every mechanic in the phone book until you find a price you're willing to pay. You can get through this rainstorm, and the grass will be much greener on the other side.

Rules You Should

Definitely Break

Do you get sick of people telling you what to do all the time? "Be here on Saturday for a last-minute marketing meeting." "Please refrain from using your cell phone." "You're being summoned for jury duty." Well here are some rules you should feel free to break—it's time to be your own woman!

Don't wear white after Labor Day. This fashion rule originated sometime between the late 1800s and the 1950s, when more and more people were entering the middle class and needed specific rules to tell them how to fit in with their new "old money" friends.[13] But this is a new day, and you are no one's fashion slave! Let your clothes express your inner self, and be bold and confident in the choices you make.

Act your age. Your life is full of responsibilities, and every once in a while you just need to let loose! Go play on a swing set, dance on a table, have a food fight. Throwing propriety to the wind might be the best thing you do for yourself today.

Eat your vegetables. While we all know it's important to maintain a balanced diet, sometimes your body has cravings that need to be met. If you've had a particularly bad day at work, don't make yourself feel guilty for eating a gallon of ice cream for dinner. Scarf down a bacon cheeseburger if you're out with the guys. Feel free to add extra whipped cream to your mocha latte every now and then. You'll be back to your salads and grilled chicken soon enough.

Don't call boys. Your mom probably drilled this one into you growing up, for fear that she'd have her little girl known as a floozy. Well, now that you're a grown woman, it's perfectly fine for you to cast your inhibitions to the wind and make a move on the man of your dreams. Be feminine, be flirtatious, and be sweet. But most important, be yourself. Let him see your personality as you hit on him—whether your style is to boldy ask him out or simply "make yourself available" for a date.

Don't run with scissors. We spend a lot of time being careful, don't we? Covering your butt on everything you do at work, making sure your husband has the story straight when your mom asks why you weren't able to come to family dinner, spending hours coming up with the perfect outfit to match the occasion . . . it gets exhausting! So let loose! Call in sick and go see a movie; schedule a solo trip to a faraway place; look up an old flame that hasn't quite burned out yet. Live dangerously. Dare to ask yourself, "What do I want?"

Awesome
International Destinations

There's a whole world out there to explore and enjoy—why not hop on a plane for your next vacation and visit another continent, another culture? Make everyone back home green with envy with your stories of international adventure or relaxation.

African game reserve. If Tiger Woods chose the Shamwari Game Reserve as the romantic setting for his marriage proposal to wife Elin Nordegren, then you know it's a place worth visiting. The luxurious private game reserve in the malaria-free Eastern Cape of South Africa is the ultimate African adventure. At Shamwari you'll experience magnificent Big Five game viewing (lions, elephants, hippos, rhinos, and leopards), lavish lodge accommodations, and one-of-a-kind spa treatments. Visit Shamwari.com to book your reservation, and enter "FIVE" in the subject line when e-mailing to reserve the Mantis Madness package—six nights free when you pay for four nights! (See their site for full details.)

Go to www gutsywomentravel.com to join a travel program designed for women, and if you enter "GWTFIVE" in the promotional code box at checkout, you'll get a $100 savings on your trip!

Chic Tokyo hotel. The Park Hotel is the best hotel for the money in Tokyo. The luxurious lobby (on the nineteenth floor of the Shiodome Tower) boasts an eleven-story, open, triangular atrium, as well as a magnificent view of the city. Park Hotel offers all amenities that you'd find in a hotel twice the price—luxury, great service—and it's much less touristy than many of its counterparts, making it the best value in Tokyo. Just remember to ask for a room with a view of the Tokyo Tower. Visit www.parkhoteltokyo.com.

Holland and Belgium river cruise. April is "Tulip Time" in Holland, so book a trip with a front-row seat for one of the most beautiful scenes in the world! And touring this landscape by river cruise allows you to experience the spectacular sights, historical attractions, cultural hot spots, and scrumptious cuisine of these delightful countries without having to pack and move from hotel to hotel. Search "European river cruises" on Google to find the perfect cruise for you.

Greece. If you dream of sparkling blue oceans and crisp white shores, take a fantasy trip to Greece! This is your chance to make those picturesque photos of beautiful beaches, colorful sunsets, and whitewashed buildings along the sea cliffs come to life. Sure you can tour the popular sites, but you can also visit a wine tasting, take a Greek cooking class, or go to an archaeological site. This is truly a destination you'll have a hard time leaving.

Austrian ski resort. If you're the athletic, sporty, but very stylish type, St. Anton, one of the most famous ski resorts in the world, is your perfect destination. It lies in "The Arlberg," the name given to five picturesque towns in Austria—an area that has always been famous for its beauty. With reliable snow extending right down to the villages, its more than 270 miles of descents are superbly prepared for all levels of ability.

Ways to Manipulate Others—
Without Getting Caught!

There comes a time when you subtly need to (and I mean subtly,) convince others of what you already know—namely, that you are right! Mastering the art of manipulation is tricky business—as soon as someone gets wise to your tactics, all is lost. Different people and different relationships call for unique, customized strategies. So here are some ideas for the key players in your life.

The man in your life. In *My Big, Fat, Greek Wedding*, Toula's mother famously says, "The man is the head [of the house], but the woman is the neck. And she can turn the head any way she wants." The key to getting your guy to come to your side is in good old-fashioned negotiations. Present your case in such a way that he discovers, on his own, the benefit of going along with your desires. Make him an offer he can't refuse.

Your boss. Are you ready for a big raise? Are you sick and tired of sitting in a cubicle next to Chatty Cathy? Are you ready to go along with the managers to make the pitch to the big account? Let your boss see the value you bring to the team. Quantify your contribution to the bottom line. Make clear the benefits to *her* when you get what you want.

Your mom/mother-in-law. Mother knows best, right? She raised you. She clearly remembers when you were nothing but a ragamuffin toddler, a pimply teenager, a dazed and confused college student—looking to her for advice and guidance. But now you know what's best for you, and you need her support. So let it be her idea. Instead of pitching her on the concepts, "think out loud" about it in front of her. Let her come to the conclusion you've already arrived at, and then thank heaven for "a great mom like her" when she arrives there.

Your friends. You get together and do the same thing every single weekend. You simply cannot take the boring routine any longer. It's time for something new! So how do you convince the crew to give up their comfortable rut? Take things into your own hands. Host an event of your liking—a wine tasting, a game night, a theme party. Surprise them with your creativity and inspire them to try something new!

Your kids. Quite possibly your children are the most stubborn, unyielding bunch of people in your entire social circle. Want to go to the park? No! Want to have some yummy lunch? No! So how do you manipulate them into obedience? Age is a factor, and the fun book *How to Con Your Kid* by David Borgenicht and James Grace gives a ton of ideas. Step one: Distract. Take their attention off whatever is making them upset. Step two: Entice. Draw them in with a tried-and-true reward. Step three: Conquer! You can now appear in public with your perfect, well-behaved children.

Unusual Ideas
for a Much-Needed Night with the Girls

When dinner and a movie aren't cutting it any longer, try one of these ideas for a fun night out with your girlfriends.

Cook at home. Call the girls and invite them over for a fun evening of cooking and eating together! Grab your favorite recipe from home, or your most recent *Cooking Light* magazine. Choose a decadent meal and dessert, make a list of all the ingredients, and make the trip to the grocery with your partner in epicurean crime. The only thing you need to do before they arrive is set a table that shouts, "Party!" to give your home a festive feeling. To make the night less expensive, you and your friends could agree to split the grocery bill. Eat, drink, and be merry!

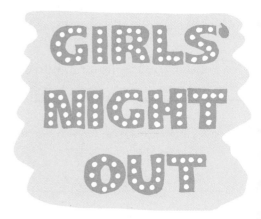

Host a charity party. Instead of indulging yourselves, why don't you and your friends "donate" an evening to charity? Choose a worthy cause, whether it be troops overseas, a local orphanage, or a homeless shelter, and ask everyone attending the party to choose something they'd like to contribute to a care package. Everyone should bring a certain quantity of her item so that you can put an equal number of packages together—sealed and addressed for you to drop off at the post office the next day. If the charity is local, make plans to visit and hand out the kits in person.

Get a room. Grab your girlfriends and your most scrumptious terry-cloth robe, and escape to a local five-star hotel for the night. Order in room service. Treat yourself to spa services. Watch a movie you know you couldn't get the men in your life to watch with you, and do what all women love to do—enjoy an evening of chatting and laughter. And sleep in! Live like the divas you are.

Chase a rock star. A killer band is in town, and you are so into the rockers. Mill around by the back entrance to the show and follow the band when they leave. Take your cameras and band tees—be a groupie. You may even get to meet your celebrity crush at a bar or their hotel if you stay hot on their trail long enough. You'll have stories and pics to show off for weeks!

Crash a party. Rent *Wedding Crashers* with your friends, then get dressed for the occasion and get ready to act the part. Do your research, and crash a wedding, a bar mitzvah, or a socialite's party. You'll get great food, fun dancing, and fabulous entertainment. You'll experience the thrill of almost getting caught. You'll laugh all night long at the hijinks you pulled!

Tips for Tackling
Stressful Situations

Find the positive. A wild roller-coaster ride is one of the most stressful situations you can put yourself in—or is it? What terrifies some people is exhilarating for others. So when you're faced with a problem you don't think you can face—like an upcoming plane trip that laughs in the face of your fear of flying—try to figure out why your coworker, your boyfriend, or your gal pal is grinning from ear to ear with excitement and embrace that aspect of your situation. Maybe they're too excited about all they'll do in their exotic destination to be worried about the travel there.

Get a reality check. No one likes to feel as if she is losing control, but we can make ourselves feel worse off than we really are when we buy into faulty perceptions of what's really going on. So take a deep breath. Count to ten. Step back and look at the situation from a new angle—ask a friend or someone unrelated to the crisis for her opinion. Maybe if you start to make some sense of it all, your stress will die down.

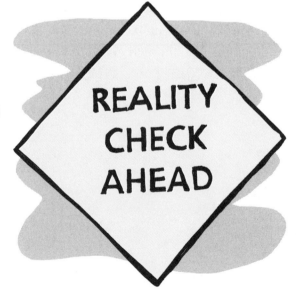

Know your stress symptoms. Some people blush, others grow pale. Some gorge on ice cream or French fries, while others lose their appetite. Stress can have a variety of effects on the GI tract, skin, and musculoskeletal and other systems. Go to www.stress.org and, under Frequently Asked Questions, click on "Effects of Stress" for a list of fifty common signs and symptoms of stress. Learn what your stress symptoms are so that you can tell when and how stress is affecting you.

Know your cure. Just as stress differs for each of us, no stress reduction strategy works for everyone. Jogging, meditating, doing yoga, or listening to music may be great for some, but when arbitrarily imposed on others, prove to be dull, boring, and potentially even more stressful. You have to find out what works best for you and practice it because you want to, not because someone tells you to.

What women want. Women's brains may be more sensitive to certain types of stress, which might explain why women are more likely to become depressed than men are. There are also hormonal differences due to the secretion of oxytocin, the "cuddling hormone." As a result, during acute stress, "fight or flight" reactions may be overpowered by a "tend and befriend" response, which means you might prefer to be comforted by a friend (i.e., marathon phone call) instead of putting the situation on the back burner (i.e., parking yourself on the couch in front of a football or video game).[14]

Ways to Give Back —
or What to Do When the TV Ads with Starving Children Start Getting to You

No idea where to start? Thanks to VolunteerMatch.org, volunteering in your local community has never been easier. Simply type in your zip code and the maximum distance you're prepared to drive to do volunteer work, choose your area of volunteer interest, and click Search. You will immediately be given a list of opportunities with the organization, location, date, and who the opportunity is "Great For" listed to help you make the choice most suited to your compassion and skills. These opportunities will include everything from hosting an exchange student to fostering an animal or doing housing repairs.

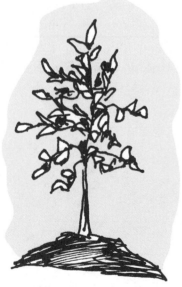

Help the elderly. Some of the most vulnerable members of our neighborhoods are senior citizens. Volunteer drivers transport the elderly to their doctor appointments or other medical services, and volunteer dispatchers schedule appointments with the drivers. A more intense need, which requires the unique ability to be able to work with terminally ill patients and their families, is for hospice volunteers who visit patients to give caregivers a break, run simple errands for the patients, and offer support during bereavement. This requires the strength to handle the loss of those you serve.

Go green. Leonardo DiCaprio's doing it. So is Cameron Diaz. And we all know about Al Gore. So get some fresh air and support an environmental project in your area: from litter cleanups to tree, flower, and bulb planting to recycling campaigns. You can also become involved in community education by teaching anyone from kids to senior citizens the importance of conserving energy, water, and waste.

Get political. Here in the USA you have a right to get involved in government's business—something not everyone on this planet is privileged to do. So take advantage of that. You can serve on local boards and committees, which are the frontlines of community participation in national politics. You just have to pick an issue you feel passionate about and get involved, whether it be the environment, health care, protection, or lifestyle issues. Don't let thoughts such as *One person can't make a difference, I don't know enough,* or *I don't have enough time* stop you.

Donate. One solution to our "buy, buy, buy" habit is to "donate, donate, donate." Clear space on your shelves—take all the books you've read and don't want to keep to the local library. Same with all the clothes you're never going to wear again or the toys your kids don't play with anymore—make a quick detour to your local Salvation Army or Goodwill. If there is a charity you would like to donate to, the safe and secure NetworkForGood.org makes it easy and convenient. All your donation records are stored and accessible anytime, making life easier at tax time.

"By the way, I ultimately do all these things for the good of mankind, right? Sometimes I don't think I come off that way."

—Lisa Weil as Paris Gellar, on needing volunteer work for her college application, *Gilmore Girls*™
© Warner Bros. Entertainment Inc.

91

Things to Remember

When You Want to Bow Out Gracefully

Be an adult. Opting for a no-show rather than having to decline an invitation is tempting, but is it worth it? The truth is you will seldom get away with it without having to give an explanation later. Your absence will arouse curiosity, and someone is sure to ask you where you were the next time he or she sees you. So, to avoid the added awkwardness of having to explain why you were not polite enough to excuse yourself, it's best just to be adult and make a call beforehand.

Honesty is not always the best policy. Even though you will feel pressure to give a detailed explanation when bowing out, it is not always necessary to give the whole truth. You have the right to simply decline an invitation without giving a reason—although this takes incredible self-control. Don't let your need to please people and fear of people disliking you tempt you into giving more of an explanation than you feel comfortable with. A simple, "I'm so sorry, we're not going to be able to make it" is all you need to say.

No need to apologize. You don't have a prior commitment or an overbooked schedule—you just don't want to do what you're being invited to do. You can still say no, and you shouldn't feel the need to apologize when you do it. You are the only one who truly knows what's best for yourself (and your family). You can be polite without making excuses or half hearted apologies.

Don't be dissuaded. Once you've made your decision to bow out, make sure you stick to it. Don't let others' persuasion change your mind. If you offer an excuse, leave it at just one. Don't go on and on with reasons you can't make it, or you may, as the old adage goes, offer "enough rope to hang yourself."

Phone or e-mail? Although sending e-mail messages is one of the many modern-day conveniences we have, remember it is not appropriate for every situation. People can be easily offended if they are sent an e-mail when they believe they should have been called. So think before you e-mail, and take the time to call when turning someone down if you think it will be better appreciated!

Body Language Signals
You Don't Want to Send (or Maybe You Do!)

I'm interested. That total jerk of a guy you had to work with on the big proposal last month is assigned to a project with you again. So how do you make sure he gets the clue that you are *not* interested in him? Make sure you stand or sit no closer than two feet away from him—keep your distance and he'll start to get the idea. Don't open up to him—keep your physical self guarded and reserved by crossing your arms or legs. Keep eye contact to a minimum. Don't mirror his body language. (This one can be hard to monitor.) Make a conscious effort not to copy what he's doing!

I'm better than you. You wouldn't dream of snapping at your boss or a potential client, or to your mom or your father-in-law. But is it possible you're being rude without even realizing it? Standing with your hands on your hips indicates aggression. Sitting with your hands clasped behind your head— typically a more "male" pose—says that you think you're superior. And touching your nose shows you doubt what they're saying is true. Beware of saying more than you mean to with these subtle gestures.

I speak two languages: Body and English.

—Mae West

94

I'm not interested. You might be on a date with a cute, cute guy, and you're nervous out of your mind. Watch out! Crossing your legs and kicking your foot ever so slightly indicates that you're bored with what he's saying. Resting your head in your hands or looking down says the same thing. But keeping your palms open shows sincerity and innocence on your part.

I'm incompetent. You've worked way past midnight every night for the last two weeks, and you've eaten gallons of ice cream to melt away the stress just getting ready for this huge project event presentation. It's understandable that your nerves are in high gear as you head into the big day. But don't let them see you sweat! Maintain a brisk walk with good posture that says, "I'm confident," not a hunched gait with your hands in your pocket that broadcasts your dejection. And be loose—locked ankles (of all things!) indicate apprehension, while steepling your fingers shows your authoritative side.

I'm completely ignorant of your culture. We all know what a raised middle finger means here in the USA, but what might be offensive in other parts of the world? If you're planning to travel, brush up on international body languages! While a thumbs-up in Kansas is a positive sign, it means "up yours" in Australia. If you wave to flag down a waiter in France, he just might spit in your food! And in Japan you had better have your shoes shined at all times. For more details, check out *Gestures: The Dos and Taboos of Body Language Around the World* by Roger E. Axtell.

Questions to Ask

Before You Get That Credit Card

Most of us get a few credit card offers in the mail every day. But when the average card-carrying American has more than $8,000 in credit card debt,[15] it's wise to be cautious in picking one. How do you weed through the junk that comes in your mail?

How do I plan to use it? Some people put all their monthly expenses on their card, and they pay it off dutifully every month. Others use it only for special purchases. And still others keep it as an "emergency only" option. How often you use your card, and how often you plan to pay it off, will affect the level of interest rate you can reasonably stand to have on your card. So be honest with yourself and plan accordingly.

What does it give me? Does your card give back for all the spending you do? If you're a big traveler, consider a card with airline miles as bonus points. If you're in the market for a new car, get a card with auto rewards. But be careful with rewards cards—you can find yourself spending more just because you're getting points back. So think twice before you buy that third Prada dress.

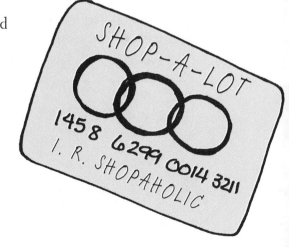

What does it cost? If the card you're signing up for has an annual fee, seriously consider running away from that offer. There are tons of free credit cards out there, so there's really no reason to spend money in addition to the interest rate.

Are they nice? The grace period on your credit card is the number of days you have until they charge you a fee for being late with your payment. If the grace period is very short—or none at all— ditch that card. There are other companies out there that will be much nicer.

> "There are times in your life when you have to do ridiculous things for money."
>
> —Lauren Graham as Lorelai Gilmore, *Gilmore Girls* ™
> © Warner Bros. Entertainment Inc.

Are they mean? If you overestimated just a bit when you bought those new sterling bangles from Tiffany, and it turns out your check this week doesn't quite cover that plus the rent, you'll want to make sure your credit card doesn't have a "penalty interest" clause in the contract. This means that the interest rate will actually rise with late payments—exponentially increasing the amount you owe your credit card company.

Experiences
Worth Having

One woman said "a bikini wax." Another said "moving to a foreign country." How do you narrow it down to just five top experiences every girl should have? "Impossible!" we cry. So, here are five spheres of your life and some suggestions for each part of yourself.

Work. Trying to make a living by doing what you love. Moving to a new city for a job. Getting fired. Going back to school. Flirting with a coworker. Speaking in public. Suggesting your idea. Doing something you can't imagine really doing for a job, just once. Standing your ground. Waiting tables. Volunteering.

Love. Saying "I love you" in public. Surviving a break up. Remarrying as a senior. Adopting a baby. Watching your kids play with their daddy. Making up! Risking it all to let him know you love him. Giving him a second chance. Waking him up in the middle of the night to live out that dream you just had. Saying "I'm sorry."

Soul. Traveling on your own. Going to confession. Studying the Bible. Talking to a counselor. Having your portrait painted. Singing in public. Journaling. Writing a book. Giving advice. Asking advice. Just crying, when that's all you need. Letting someone in and truly trusting that person. Living sustainably.

Body. Having a baby without an epidural. Getting a massage. Getting a bikini wax. Getting plastic surgery. Skydiving. Training for a marathon. Taking Sundays off. Eating organic food. Flaunting it. Accepting a compliment without an excuse.

Money. Making a risky investment. Starting a business. Saving 10 percent. Tithing. Giving too much to a person in need. Accepting a gift without pretenses. Paying off a mortgage. Telling a lawyer no. Spending money on something luxurious.

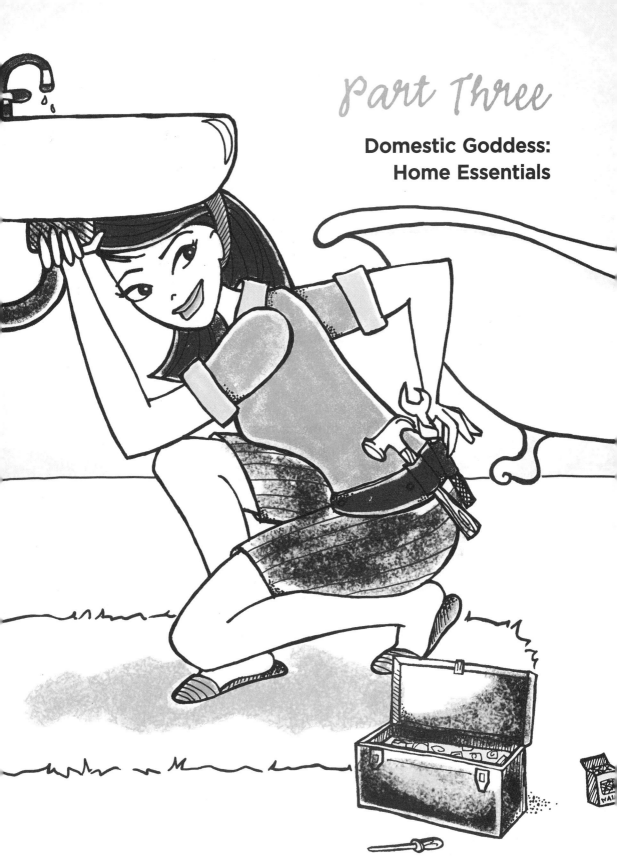

Part Three

**Domestic Goddess:
Home Essentials**

Ways to Make 5

Your House Look Clean . . . Fast

You have just received the dreaded phone call: "We're on our way. Is it okay if we stop by for a minute to say hi?" While you're (maybe) excited to see your friends, in-laws, or neighbors, you would have appreciated some advance notice! So here's how to do a quick cleanup when you only have a couple of minutes before your guests arrive.

Floor them. Do a quick vacuum of your main thoroughfares. Sprucing up your high-traffic areas can have a dramatic effect on the illusion of clean carpets. If you have hardwoods, just take your area rugs outside for a quick shakedown.

Is that new? Fluff the pillows on your couches or armchairs. Not only is it more comfortable for your guests to sit on, it looks cleaner when it's more neatly arranged. Spray a quick blast of Febreeze or another air-purifying spray if you have pets that like to sit on the couch. And if you have an extra minute, you might run the vacuum over the couch and under the seat cushions as well.

It only takes a spark. A freshly lit candle with a clean scent, such as linen or citrus, will take the odor out of your kitchen. You'll not regret the salmon you had last night quite so much with a pretty, aromatic flame hiding your leftover scents. (And take the trash out if you have stinky kitchen smells lingering.)

Flush. Do a quick Pine-Sol rinse on your toilet bowls. Guests will think you live in a state of perpetual spick-and-span. Always keep a bottle of this cleaner in each bathroom. When guests are expected, pour in a bit and give it a quick brush. Let it sit for a minute before flushing, and your bathroom will smell like you spent hours scouring it.

Mirror, mirror. Don't forget to freshen up yourself. Stop by the mirror on the way to the door and primp up your hair, refresh your lipstick, and straighten your shirt. Remember, you're trying to make them think the house is always this clean, so don't let them see you sweating and panting after your whirlwind cleanup!

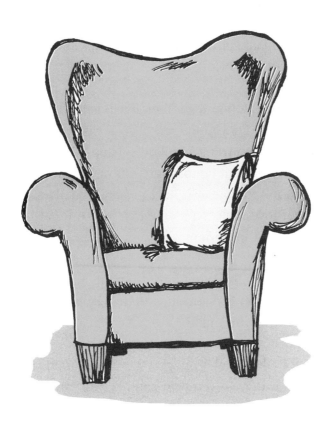

Secrets for Throwing
a Killer Birthday Party

Phyllis Cambria, award-winning event planner, co-owner of PartyPlansPlus.com, and coauthor of several party-planning books, including *The Complete Idiot's Guide to Throwing a Great Party*, says, "Parties should be as much fun for the host as they are for the guest of honor and guests. A little bit of thought, a sense of humor, and some preplanning can go a long way to making the experience one you'll want to repeat again and again." Here are her tips for easy entertaining for birthdays or any special occasion.

The theme's the thing. Choosing a theme will actually help you with your hosting duties because it allows you to focus your ideas on the food, decorations, and entertainment rather than using a scattershot approach. When choosing one for a birthday, reflect the guest of honor's interests or hobbies. It can be anything from a preferred vacation spot to a favorite TV show. Whether it's a hobby or food the guest of honor loves, select a theme that lets your pal know you planned the party especially for him or her.

Budgets—big or small. You don't have to spend a fortune to have a great celebration. Just plan your budget and stick to it. While smaller budgets may require a little more work—you might have to cook instead of having food catered or create the décor from scratch rather than buying ready-made decorations—you *can* make smaller budgets work to your advantage. Simply gather family and friends to help, and you can have a "party before the party"! On the other hand, if money is not an issue and your time is limited, it's loads of fun to hire (the right) party professionals who can help you to fulfill your theme dream. You can just write the check and take the bows.

Inviting ideas. Invitations are your guests' first clue as to the type of party they will be attending. Make your invitation speak as loudly as the party itself so that your guests get excited about the birthday bash in advance. Get creative with art, gadgets, and goodies that can be incorporated into the invitation details instead of trying to jam all of your info on one of those fill-in-the-blank ho-hum invitations.

Guests don't like to guess. When planning your party, think like a guest. Consider every step your guests will have to take when coming to your event. Does the invitation contain all of the details they need besides the normal "who, what, when, where, and why"? Did you include RSVP details, directions, and dress code suggestions? Mentally walk through everything your guest will experience from the moment they arrive to when they leave. Where will they park? Where will they hang their coats? What will they eat? What type of entertainment will they have? How will they be greeted? How will the party end? By thinking it through from a guest's perspective, you'll create the party like a pro.

Party "oops." It happens to everyone. No matter how well you plan, things can sometimes go wrong. The best thing to do is to keep a sense of humor and a level head. Dinner burned? Bring in takeout. The power goes out? Light some candles. Spilled wine? Cover it with a damp cloth and deal with it later. The point is if you don't overreact, neither will your guests. Think of it this way, the bigger the "oops," the more likely it is to become a great party story that will get funnier with each retelling in the months and years to come.

How to Be the Perfect Hostess—
or at Least Look Like One!

Greet them. Well, it's unlikely that you wouldn't greet your guests at the door, since they wouldn't be able to get in otherwise, but there's more to it than just letting them in. Be excited to see them. Greet them warmly. Be specific in your greeting—comment on your girlfriend's new shirt, your mom's new haircut, and so on. And walk to the door and wave as they leave; let them know you were glad to have them and are sad to see them go.

Feed them. Have a treat prepared, or buy one and pass it off as your own. Set it out on a nice dish on the kitchen counter for them to snack on while you hang out or while they're waiting for dinner if you're planning to eat together. An easy savory idea is to spread pepper-jack pimento cheese over toasted baguette slices and heat them in the oven for fifteen minutes. These make a yummy appetizer that goes a long way.

Be positive. No one likes to hang out with Debbie Downer, so don't fill your conversation with depressing topics. Avoid talking about the newly ousted pastor at your church, your cousin's mother-in-law who just got bad news from the doctor, or your neighbor who seems to have fallen off the wagon . . . again.

Document their visit. Buy a hostess diary or a blank journal for guests to sign when they come over. You can get a really formal one that functions as a pretty centerpiece. Or you can get any blank journal to use more casually—guests can write funny comments or answer questions you have written in, such as, "What's your dream vacation?"

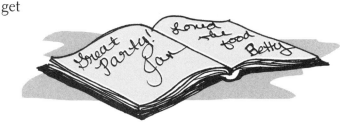

Pay attention. Do you know the biblical story of Mary and Martha? Martha's running around like crazy getting food on the table, keeping drinks filled, and making sure the entertainment is all set in place, while Mary is simply sitting around with their guests, enjoying the company of the guest of honor, Jesus. When Martha complains that Mary's not helping enough, Jesus tells her that Mary's doing the better thing—just hanging out and spending time with people. So if you tend to stress out and panic when you have people over, just focus on the fact that they'll remember the conversation more than the origami napkins you folded or the exact flavors of the ten-spice chili you served for dinner.

Things You Need to Know

About Your Neighbors . . . So You Don't Have to Spy on Them

"It's a beautiful day in the neighborhood, a beautiful day for a neighbor . . ." Mr. Rogers sang these words to many of us every day growing up, but do we really believe them now that we're living in the global village? How well do you know the people living next door to you? Do you know their names? Would you even recognize their faces if you had to pick them out of a lineup? Here are some ways to stay current on the folks next door.

The basics. Ask their names, even if you've lived there for a year and know, you should remember what they are. Write them down later and keep them on your fridge or desk—just remember to stash it away should they come in for a visit! And from then on, use their names when you say hello. Saying the name actually helps imprint it in your mind.

Their criminal records. Do a quick search for your street and zip code on www.familywatchdog.us to find out if you have any sex offenders living in your neighborhood. This is a great site that not only tells you where registered sex offenders live, but shows you their mug shots too! Learn their faces, and if you have kids, figure out a way to discreetly tell them about "stranger, danger." As GI Joe said, "Knowing is half the battle." And if there's a particular person in your community who seems suspicious, consider doing a background check on him or her!

Their pet peeves. Do your neighbors hate it when people mow the lawn at seven o'clock in the morning, and do they get angry when dogs poop in their yards? Do you hate it when the people in the apartment next to you watch *Deal or No Deal* at deafening volumes or when they leave their bags of trash outside their front door to take to the dumpster in the morning? Know what annoys your neighbors, and let them know what drives you nuts. You can find a clever way to work it into a conversation, or you can just ask them their pet peeves and tell them yours in return.

It's been awhile. Have you not seen your neighbor in a *long* time? Has her car not moved in a few weeks? Call the landlord to check on her if you think there's a chance something might be wrong.

The advantage of knowing them. Getting to know your neighbors can have hidden benefits. Does it turn out that the guy next door owns the café you go to once a week? Let him know it's your favorite spot, and maybe he'll give you the "friends and family" discount. Are you a freelance editor with a publisher living next door? Let her know your skills, and she can put you in circulation at her company. The more you let your neighbors know about yourself, the more you might find ways to benefit from their connections!

Recipes You Need to Memorize
to Impress Your Friends and Family

Did you know that in the nineteenth and twentieth centuries many recipes were written as rhyming poems to make them easier for homemakers to memorize? You don't need to memorize recipes today—that's what your custom cookbook cabinet and kitchen computer station are for. Or do you? Here are some recipes that are worth memorizing—even if only to impress!

Cocktail bar. Next time you have the girls over for drinks, wouldn't it be impressive if you could whip up refreshing cocktails from memory? It just won't look as cool if you're studying a mix recipe as you timidly measure out the necessary ingredients. So memorize a few fancy cocktail recipes, or even tweak your favorite to give it your signature flavor.

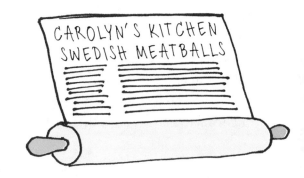

Domestic goddess. It is good to memorize at least one recipe for an impressive entree so you can pull out all the stops on vacation with friends or if you get a last-minute call while you're running errands that your husband is bringing his boss home for dinner. Pick a recipe that isn't too complicated with dozens of ingredients that are hard to find. But, at the same time, the recipe can't be too simple either—it has to be able to impress the most domestic mother-in-law!

Dessert queen. If you don't feel confident enough to make dinner for the friends or family you are staying with—for fear of it not turning out right—then claim the dessert course! A simple, elegant, and delicious dessert like chocolate cups with whipped cream filling that can be made in about five minutes (but needs to be prepared about two hours before the meal) is perfect. When your guests have finished eating, all you'll need to do is fill the cups and garnish with a mint sprig or drizzle of liqueur.[1]

Coffee shop. An impressive hospitality trick is to offer guests a choice of coffees after dinner. Not a variety of flavors but a coffee shop choice of an espresso, cappuccino, Americano, or latte. You want to be able to chat with your guests while effortlessly fulfilling the "orders," so there will be no place for checking a recipe. All you need to make these coffees is an espresso machine, which also steams and froths milk.

Food to go. It's the question you hate to ask: Can I bring something? But if you travel in the casual social circles where potluck dinners are common—most likely if you're a girl in the South—you had better be prepared to have a recipe that's easy to make ahead and one that travels easily. Pick a side dish you enjoy eating a lot, and perfect the execution of it. Make it one that's not too sloshy in the car and one you won't get sick of eating every time you go to dinner at a friend's house.

Things You Should Drop
Like a Bad Habit

Does your life feel too full—as if it's about to overflow or even explode? Less debt, a tidier home, and no more junk e-mail could create a little more order in your life. But what about being able to wake up in the morning and look forward to the day ahead without dreading the overdue obligations on your to-do list? It's time to recognize the "junk" in your life.

Guilt. New Year's Day. Birthdays. These days should be celebrations of the past year, but instead, most of us find ourselves wallowing in the guilt of unaccomplished goals. Imagine waking up in the morning without worrying about the chores and obligations you have put off. Could it be because of a desire for perfection—a faulty image of what our lives should be—that we're letting guilt rule our lives? It's time to throw petty guilt out and replace it with optimism. Meditate on the positives in your past and in each new day you face. Time passes by so quickly; enjoy it before it's gone!

Spam. No, not the canned "meat" in your grandma's kitchen cupboard—well, okay, maybe toss that out too. But you *need* to get rid of the junk e-mail you didn't ask for that relentlessly fills up your inbox daily. Never buy anything from an unsolicited e-mail advertisement, and never reply to spam. If you do this, you'll only confirm that your e-mail address is active, making your address valuable and likely to be sold to other spammers. If this has already happened, there's little you can do to stop it short of switching to a new e-mail address. You can add spammers to your junk e-mail list (which is a bit time consuming), or if you use a Mac, you can hit shift-apple-B to bounce an unwanted e-mail back to the sender, making it look like it was sent to an invalid e-mail address.[2]

The dog. Has that cute, cuddly puppy turned into a menace you could do without in your life? Do you fantasize about giving that little bundle of fur a good kick to the curb? If your heart is steely cold toward him, you can pursue the path of finding Fido a new home. However, the most reasonable option is to drop your dog's bad habits instead. Most common behavior problems can be easily solved in training classes. Give your pet another chance!

Clutter. Getting in the right frame of mind to throw out *stuff* requires brutal honesty. When was the last time you used it? Does it have true sentimental value, or are you just making excuses? Can you sell it on eBay? Do you know someone who could use it? Ask yourself these questions about everything in your closet, pantry, and attic. And put everything in a keep, sell, give away, or trash pile. It's time to be heartless: feeling guilty about getting rid of that panini maker your great-aunt Erma gave you when you're on a no-carb diet makes no sense. Have patience: making these piles will not be pretty, but it is the first step toward the near-euphoric feeling of order and accomplishment.

Debt. If you have a lot of debt, budgets may not be your strong suit. But they're the first step you have to take in climbing out of that dark hole of financial stress. Make a list of everyone you owe money to, smallest to biggest, and knock them off one at a time. You'll feel a great sense of accomplishment in checking those names off one by one. And cut up those credit cards—the last thing you need on your mind is temptation to spend more money!

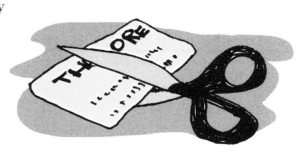

Things to Look for
When Renting an Apartment

GAIL: As you can see, it's a bit of a fixer-upper.
KIRSTEN: That's one way to put it.
SANDY: Who are you kidding, Gail? This place is a first-class
   dump. And I like it!

—from *The OC* ™

Know what you want. The most important thing for you to do before you start looking for a place is to know what you are looking for. Do you need a two-bedroom in an affordable neighborhood? Do you want a big complex with an active social network—wireless lobbies and happy hours? Do you need a safe area so you can jog alone at night? Do you want to play tennis every afternoon? This will help you narrow your search and will save you tons of time before you even get started.

Consider your budget. First things first—there's no point wasting time looking at $1,500 per month apartments when all you can afford is $500 per month. Setting your budget will help you figure out what part of town to look in, how many bedrooms to ask for, and even if you need to find a roommate to go in on a tonier apartment with you!

Location, location, location. Do you want to be within five minutes of your office? Do you have a favorite restaurant or bar or store you want to live near? Are there train tracks running right behind your bedroom window, or is there a smelly fish market across the street?

You can find an apartment almost anywhere in town, so consider the important location factors before you sign on the dotted line.

Understand the legalese. Make sure you know exactly what you're getting into once you find the perfect apartment. How long is your lease? And what happens if you have to break it early? Are pets allowed—even if you don't own a pet, you should ask if you want to avoid being woken up by barking dogs or living with constantly itchy eyes from the cat who lived there before you. This is also the time to find out if the rent includes any utilities, if you get a security deposit back when you leave, and if there are any cleaning fees upon moving out.

Who's in charge? Find out at the outset who is responsible for what and how problems are handled. Who do you call when the toilet breaks—the landlord or the plumber? Can you paint the walls in your bedroom? Ask if you can get the names and phone numbers of a couple of current renters, and call them to see how happy they are with the responsiveness of the maintenance staff.[3]

Fun and Creative Shower Ideas—
for Weddings and Babies, not Personal Hygiene!

Hosting a shower can be a pain in the neck, but it's a great way to honor your sister, your best friend, or that girl from the office whom you barely know but who doesn't have any friends to throw her a party to celebrate this huge event in her life. So how do you plan a party that is fun, memorable, and meaningful to the guest of honor? Here are some fresh ideas for your stale party brain!

Honor her. A wedding or baby shower is the perfect time for you to say all those deep, meaningful sentiments that are a little out of place when you're just shopping or catching a movie. So take a few minutes to think about what the guest of honor means to you—what do you love about her, and how will that make her a great wife or mother? Write it down in your card, or if you're super gutsy, deliver a speech to kick things off. She'll likely remember the things you said more than any of the gifts she gets.

Test her. Anyone entering the world of marriage or parenthood for the first time likely thinks she has it all together but is actually totally clueless about what is in store for her! You'll all get a few laughs if you poke some fun at the things that will blindside her in the near future. Hold a diaper-changing competition, a baby-food taste-test

challenge, a last-minute-dinner-for-the-boss quiz, or a one-minute race to see who can come up with the most excuses to get out of sex!

Pamper her. If your friend lives a busy, harried, stressed-out life, or if she's a total princess who loves to indulge, plan a luxurious party full of pampering for all the guests. Whether it's her last few weeks of sleep before a screaming infant interrupts her nights or her last month of solitude and silence at home before a man moves in, plan a party complete with spa treatments, gourmet food, high-end décor, or special guests she didn't expect to get to spend time with—whatever floats her boat.

Humor her. If your friend is the life of the party, loves a good laugh, and has a great sense of humor, plan a party that caters to her personality. Organize a "newlywed" game by asking her fiancé or husband questions beforehand—and videotape his answers—that she'll have to answer in front of the group. Have prizes for each answer—a "naughty" bag and a "nice" bag, depending on if she gets it right or wrong.

Shower yourself. If you have a special event coming up in your life—and people will want to buy you presents for it—create a registry! You don't have to be getting married or having a baby to have all the fun. Tons of people will want to congratulate you when you graduate from school, buy a house, or move to a new city. A registry makes life simpler for your friends and fans—and helps you get your new life off to a great start!

Things You Need
to Keep in Your Fridge

Frozen meals. For those hectic days when you don't have the energy to prepare dinner or even go out for a meal, you will be glad to have something in your freezer that is fast, healthy, and tasty. Yes, there is such a thing as a healthy frozen meal. In a study for *Prevention* magazine, nutritionist Janis Jibrin, RD, picked entrees that had great flavor, a third of the recommended daily calories, and were low in saturated fats. Go to www.prevention.com/pdf/pvn_frozenmeals.pdf to see her results.

Baking soda. An opened box of baking soda in your refrigerator and freezer will absorb the stinky odor from your leftover tuna melt or super-green power smoothie. You should replace the box every three months—so you might want to write the date on the side. And you don't need to invest in those fancy versions they make just for this purpose. A basic box is just as effective and much cheaper.

To be prepared is half the victory.

—*Miguel de Cervantes Saavedra*

Healthy cravings. There's nothing wrong with snacking; it's what we snack on that can be a problem. Eating several small meals a day—every two or three hours—is a good way to keep your energy level up . . . if you eat healthy snacks, that is. For those carb cravings, stock plain popcorn, which you can drizzle with a little butter or margarine without trans fats, and keep your refrigerator stocked with fruit and smoothie ingredients for that sweet tooth.

Frozen corn. When you need an ice pack and don't have time to drive to the store to buy one, grab a packet of frozen corn. It's a great alternative to those expensive brand-name, one-time-use packs at the drugstore. Another option: double bag a zippered bag partially filled with dishwashing detergent, *or* use a solution of one part rubbing alcohol and two parts water, and freeze it![4]

Wine and gourmet crackers. Nothing creates an atmosphere of sophistication and comfort like the offer of a glass of wine. Always keep a bottle of white wine chilling in the fridge and a bottle of red and a box of fancy crackers in the cupboard to offer guests. You never know when you may want to invite someone over after work, after a movie, or when the man in your life might do so without giving you much warning.

Questions to Ask
Your Prospective Pet-sitter

If you thought hiring a pet-sitter was as easy as paying the neighbor's kid a few dollars to feed and walk your dog, think again. Here are some key points to consider and to ask your prospective pet-sitter before you assign the important job of caring for and controlling the activities of your beloved pet.

"Do you know pet CPR?" Well . . . expecting your pet-sitter to know how to do pet CPR on your furry friend, as precious as she is to you, may be a bit much to ask. But, of course, it's a definite bonus if you can find one who is in fact that serious about her job. Don't settle for someone who doesn't recognize that Muffy is actually a part of the family, not "just a pet."

"What will the "living" arrangements be?" Your annual beach vacation will be all the more relaxing if you have the peace of mind of knowing what your pet's living conditions are while you're away. If he is going to be staying at the pet-sitter's, find out if he will be confined in a crate or if there are other animals there you know your dog will hate. Also, is there room for Fido's favorite bed? Will he be fed his regular food? Make sure the person has arrangements you're comfortable with before dropping off your pet.

"What will your pet's walking routine be?" If you're interviewing a petsitter to watch your dog, find out if he will be taking other dogs out with yours when he walks them, and whether he will be walking in your neighborhood or transporting your pet somewhere else. Another good idea is to have him come to your house and accompany you on a walk around the block with your dog. You can observe how he handles your pet and whether or not your dog likes him.

"What responsibility are you willing to assume?" No one wants to have to think about it, but if the worst should happen it's best to know what level of responsibility your pet-sitter is willing to take. In most cases there will be no way of knowing or proving whether she is responsible, so it is best to let her know ahead of time what will be the fair arrangement should an accident happen. Make sure you hire someone with insurance to protect himself—and you—if an unfortunate event does arise. This should include bodily injury in case Fido bites or scratches anyone while out on a walk; property damage coverage for any damage that may be caused to your own or other's property while you are away; and protection in case your pet is injured or worse while you're gone.[5]

"Do you have any references I can call?" Just as you would if you werehiring a babysitter, it's always a good idea to ask a prospective pet-sitter for references and to actually call them. Precious Fido is your fluffy "baby," right?

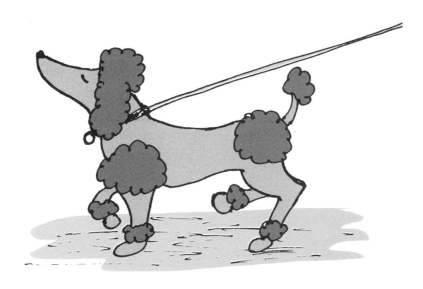

Things You Need to Know

Before You Buy a House

Buying a house is a huge step for anyone, and the amount of information you *don't* know can be overwhelming. So instead of enrolling in a real-estate class or training as a mortgage banker, ask yourself these five questions for a painless home-buying experience.

What do you want? Take a few minutes to imagine your dream home. What does it look like? What special features does it have? Are you lusting after a laundry room or a spectacular view of downtown? Do you have to have three bedrooms, or would it be better to have a spectacular office with built-in bookshelves? Do you want a fence, a pool, a high-tech media room? If you're buying a house with someone else, have that person make a list, too, and give them separately to your agent.

What can you buy? Before you start visiting homes all across town, find out what exactly is in your price range. How do you know? Get prequalified for a home loan. You can do this online at LendingTree.com, or you can make an appointment at your local bank to talk one-on-one with a mortgage lender. Having this done before you look helps a lot—this way you can go ahead and make a solid offer when you visit a house or condo you love!

Where do you want to live? Considering location is critical when you're buying real estate. Not only does it affect your day-to-day life—How long is the commute to work? Is there a grocery nearby? How far is it from your friends and family?—but it will affect your ability to resell the property later. So make sure you're not paying too much for the area. Or if you're planning to rent the house out after you move on to bigger and better things, think about whether it's in an area that you can easily find renters in.

What will you need to fix? Do you love historic homes but don't have a single DIY bone in your body? Or have you found the perfect loft condominium but it doesn't have the exposed brick walls you were hoping for? Calculate the costs (and likelihood) of renovations into your overall price of the purchase. And have an inspection done on the home before you buy—this can become your personal to-do list for home maintenance once you move in.

Who do you trust? Find an agent who comes highly recommended by your friends or coworkers. Learn the details of your friends' experience buying a house—not all real estate agents were created equally! Did their agent head to the beach on closing day? Did they delay in returning calls—to their clients and potential buyers? Or were they spectacularly attentive—making helpful suggestions and giving thoughtful insights throughout the process. And once you decide on an agent, trust her to walk you through the home-buying journey. Constantly second-guessing her will make the experience miserable for everyone involved.[6]

Things to Do When
You Desperately Need to Organize Your Closets

MARIE: I don't lose things, Frank. I'm organized.
FRANK: Not organized—insane! She's got a shoe box labeled
"pieces of string too small to use."
—from *Everybody Loves Raymond*

Prepare. It's a real pain in the neck to get started on a project like closet cleaning and then have to stop halfway through. So set aside at least three to four hours, and make sure you have access to a full-length mirror (you'll be trying on everything). Buy matching hangers, and have ones that are made for specific types of clothing—pants, dresses, skirts.

Get messy. Dump your entire closet out onto the floor of your bedroom and be relentless. The shoe with the broken heel that you never got around to fixing—trash! The flannel shirts from high school—dump them. You will be surprised at how much you can get rid of and how little you really need. If you haven't worn it in a year, it's pretty safe to give it away. And limit yourself to only three items of sentimental value.

Divide and conquer. Divide the clothes you have kept into business, casual, and evening wear. And if you are one of the lucky ones who actually go on those long-promised Caribbean vacations, make a pile for vacation wear. By organizing your clothes this way, you will know what section to turn to in a snap. When you are dividing your wardrobe, pay attention to your "comfort zones"—do you have sixteen white button-down shirts? Seven pairs of black pants? Make a mental note to avoid those items when you shop. Stepping outside your comfort zone will help you expand your wardrobe and experiment with other styles.

Be ruthless! It may help to have a very honest friend come by for this part of the journey toward organization. Try on *everything*! Make sure it still fits well, with no pulls, tears, or unseemly tucks or threads. If it's too tight, too bright, or just plain outdated, even if it's in mint condition, get rid of it! Sell anything in great shape on eBay, make notes of what you need to replace, and go shopping! And commit to make any needed trip to the dry cleaner's or alterations shop within a week.

Mission accomplished. Now that you've kept only the best of the best, it's time to put it all away. Hang pants, skirts, shirts, thick sweaters, and jackets. Fold heavy items such as jeans and very delicate items such as undergarments and cashmere or other loose knits, that will lose their shape if hung. Arrange your clothes according to business, casual, and evening wear.[7]

Decorating Tips
for Your Small—Uh, Tiny—Apartment

Trying to make a small space both stylish and practical can seem overwhelming. So if you live in an apartment that makes your cubicle feel spacious, take a few of these tips into consideration when you're setting up house.

Go high-tech. To save space in your kitchen and laundry room, invest in some high-tech appliances, such as an under-the-counter refrigerator or a dishwasher drawer. Go wireless to clean up the cord clutter. And download your music to your laptop or iPod and sell all those CDs.

Lighten up. The worst thing about having a small apartment is feeling cramped and claustrophobic when you're inside. So make an effort to keep your windows super clean to let in more light. Install some track lighting and aim it at the walls to create a feeling of expanse in your space. Put high-quality lighting fixtures inside your closets so you can find things quickly. And use full-spectrum lightbulbs to create a sense of energy.

Spend wisely. Instead of filling your house with clutter, by a few nice pieces for both decoration and practical use. Invest in high-quality cookware and linens. Hang one large art piece on the wall instead of many smaller mismatched frames. Drawing attention to these luxury items will make the place seem high-end despite its size, and you'll feel pampered even though you're perhaps a bit cramped.

Coordinate colors. The larger the variety of colors and patterns you use in your apartment, the smaller it will feel. So pick a monochromatic color scheme—go tone on tone with your upholstery and draperies. Use soft, warm colors and cool shades on the walls to make your room feel more open—avoid bright or dark paint. And coordinate the furniture with the wall color so that you won't feel as if your space is interrupted by your stuff.

Fill it up. People who entertain a lot tend to keep their apartments more organized and tidy, so don't be shy just because you're space is small. Think of it as intimate—your guests will actually socialize and converse better in close quarters.[8]

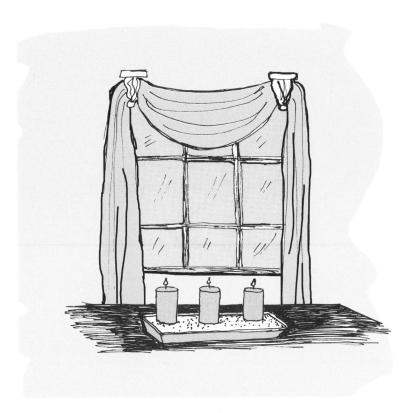

Basics of a
Beautiful Garden

Garden close to home. The less frequently you visit your garden, the less you'll maintain it. If you're just starting out, put an herb garden in your kitchen. If you're more determined, put a flower bed somewhere between your front door and your driveway, and you'll pass by it twice a day. That flower bed will be carefully tended, weed-free, and immaculately deadheaded. The further your garden is from air-conditioning and lemonade, the more weeds it will have.

Do a little each day. Even if it's only five minutes, make some time in your life each day for a bit of gardening. Instead of watching the news with your morning coffee, carry your mug out to the garden. You'll miss the crime blotter and the death toll, but you'll get news of first blossoms and nestlings taking flight. You'll be able to catch the weed seedlings before they set seed and pinch off the aphid-infested leaves before they spread.

The greatest gift of the garden is the restoration of the five senses.

—Hanna Rion

Do your research. A plant in the wrong spot is a waste of your time and effort. It will either die young, fail to reach its potential, or require constant maintenance. A poorly planned garden will be a source of frustration. The best gardeners have extensive libraries and journals full of sketches and notes. Don't know where to start? You need look no further than HGTV.com, one of the most fabulous gardening Web sites around.

Invest in infrastructure. Gardening is all about the plants. But keep in mind that when you're first getting started, plants can be had on the cheap. You can start things from seed, take cuttings from a neighbor, or divide perennials. Infrastructure, on the other hand, is pricey but gives a lot of bang for the buck. Do you need compost, raised beds, terraced slopes, or good-quality tillage tools? Spend money on infrastructure and your gardening will be a pleasure. Ignore it and you will soon trade in your trowel for a tennis racket.

Train, don't prune. Training plants is the art of directing growth where you want it to go, rather than removing it from where you don't. It's easy enough to tell if a branch is going to grow in the wrong direction. Take it out when it's small, before you have to do corrective pruning.[9]

Ways to Make

Your Home Feel Martha Stewart-Stylish

It doesn't take much to turn a well-decorated room into a cluttered mess. And what do you do if you have no idea where to even start in fixing up your personal spaces? Here are some easy tips to make you look like a style diva.

Have great cookware. To make your kitchen look like one of those gourmet, gleaming rooms in design magazines, invest in some high-end cookware and display it prominently! Copper pots and pans are beautiful but require a lot of upkeep. And many famous chefs are designing their own lines of cooking essentials in sleek stainless steel and bold colors. Pick a line that fits your personality, and then keep it in good condition—be sure to follow the manufacturer's instructions on usage and cleaning.

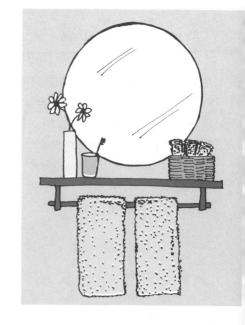

Declutter the bathroom. Too often we walk into a bathroom to face a sea of toothpaste, face cleaners, and makeup. Don't think of your bathroom as a big closet with a toilet in it; instead, make strategic decorating decisions for this potentially very relaxing room! Buy a set of matching canisters to hold the items you use daily but don't want to look at all the time. Style the space with shells, smooth stones, or flowers—something that soothes and relaxes you while you take a long bath or linger over your primping. And don't be afraid to hang some art on the walls. Whether it's a favorite painting or a stylized photo of the kids in the bathtub, just make it personal.

Make room to relax. You need a place in your home or apartment to get away from all the stress of your life and relax, and the best place to do this is the bedroom. To avoid fitful sleep and restless thoughts running through your head, keep this space limited in its "function." So, keep it TV-free, or at least have a cabinet where you can hide the TV when you're ready to rest. Don't keep piles of work next to your bed; instead, keep your favorite magazines and books in a stylish basket. And have plenty of photos of loved ones or favorite places surrounding you—you'll feel the love they generate in you as you recharge for the next day.

Love your workspace. Chances are your cubicle at work is not quite as stylish as *Ugly Betty's* offices at *Mode*. But even if your boss refuses to buy the fun floral filing folders and goes with plain manila instead, you can style your home office however you want! Get in back-to-school mode and shop for fun office accessories online at sites like SeeJaneWork.com or Target.com. Get a flat-screen monitor to save precious space, and avoid halogen bulb lamps that transport you back to cubicle-land. Use a xenon bulb lamp instead.

Show off your style. Your guests will develop their sense of your style from the spaces where they spend the most time at your home—probably your living room. To keep a Martha Stewart–clean look in your entertaining space, resist the urge to put all your favorite pieces there. Pick a few favorites and really play up their prominence. Arrange your furniture so that conversation will flow easily—make chairs and sofas face each other, not the TV. And limit your color palette to keep the room from feeling too chopped up.

Ways to Fake It
as a Domestic Goddess

Do you find your self sprawled on the couch at night, lustily flipping through your favorite obsession? No, not those syrupy romance novels, handbooks to your other secret desire—*Martha Stewart Living*, *Domino*, and *ReadyMade*. You long to be a domestic diva, but you have a hard time boiling an egg, much less making creme brulée! If this is you, then here are some tips to faking your way through domestic bliss.

—Kate Etue

Future gourmet chef. If you want your friends begging for your recipes, your first step toward becoming chef extraordinaire is to buy a gourmet cookbook or magazine. Stick to mac and cheese during the week, and save the time, effort, and expense of gourmet cooking for impressing your dinner guests. When your friends or family compliment your meal, tell them you're in training as a gourmet chef (you can leave out the self-taught part!). Someone may even want to join you in your quest for greatness. (For inspiration, pick up a copy of *Julie and Julia* by Julie Powell. It's the funny and compelling memoir of Julie's yearlong goal of cooking every recipe in Julia Child's landmark *Mastering the Art of French Cooking* cookbook.)

Maid to order. Even if you can't always eat off the floors in your house, you never want guests to see you living in filth! The best way to keep your house neat and clean is to take a few minutes at the beginning of each day to straighten and tidy. After you eat breakfast, make sure everything is put back in its place, the floors are swept if there's noticeable dirt on them. And do a quick wipe-down of the guest bathroom to hide any grime or odors.

Suzy homemaker. If you're going for the best-all-around, does-it-all reputation as a domestic diva, you'll always have something homemade to offer your guests—whether it's cookies, lemonade, or fruit tea. The good impression that a made-from-scratch refreshment makes far outweighs the short amount of time it takes to prepare. Another easy tip: a flourishing potted plant at the front door and some herbs growing in the kitchen are clever ways to distract attention from the fact that you don't do any gardening.

Top designer. You can recognize a stylish room instantly—and even worse, a tacky one—but when you're staring at blank walls and plain carpet, you have no idea where to start! If this sounds like you, it's time to bring in backup. Call in the help of a gifted friend, or shamelessly copy the décor of rooms you like in magazines. Start with the rooms guests are most likely to see when visiting—the entrance, guest bathroom, dining room, kitchen, and living room—if you're on a budget.

Hostess with the mostest. If you've ever decided to host a party and then dreaded the thought of entertaining a lot of guests who don't know each other, you are in need of some quick solutions to faking it as a hostess. First things first, and it may sound simple, but a bright smile and enthusiastic greeting goes a long way toward making your guests feel welcome and comfortable in your home. Also, take a few minutes before everyone shows up and see if you can think of anything they have in common. Then, all you will need to do ismention these common interests when you introduce them and let their conversation take off!

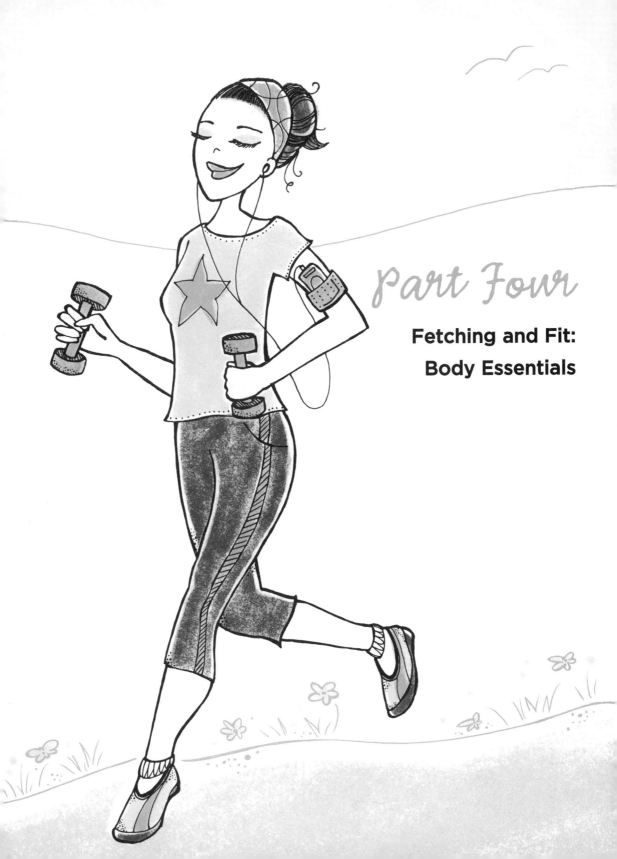

Part Four

Fetching and Fit:
Body Essentials

Vitamins You
Should Be Eating

Drink your OJ. Orange juice, best when from concentrate—weird, huh?—is a great source of folic acid. This is the penultimate prevention prescription. It helps your body produce normal red blood cells and even may help prevent stroke, colon, and breast cancer. And if you've got baby fever, load up on the folic acid. It helps a baby's spine and brain develop correctly. If you're already drinking all the OJ you can take, get some folic acid elsewhere by eating asparagus, broccoli, black beans, or peanuts.[1]

Cheese it up. Women need calcium for strong bones—you don't want to be hunched over and suffering from severe osteoporosis when you're older, do you? So add some cheese on that burger. Drink your milk. Have some yogurt for breakfast. And if you're tired of dairy, grab some almonds or hazelnuts, dried apricots or figs, or throw some tofu in that stir-fry.[2]

Steak out. If you find yourself feeling tired and irritated, don't immediately blame your boss or your kids—it might be a lack of iron in your diet. Lean red meat is a great source of iron, which you need for healthy blood and muscles. So fix steak and eggs for breakfast for a double dose of iron. Or if your not a meat eater, fill your plate with dark leafy veggies such as kale, spinach, or savoy cabbage. And

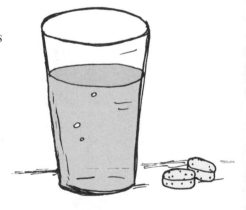

136

if it's your sweet tooth you want to please, grab some licorice to get that iron intake.[4]

Add some color. One good way to make sure you're eating well is to put a rainbow on every plate—dish up some nice red, orange, and green veggies alongside that white or red meat and your carbs. And those bright colors are often a good source of vitamin C, which is an antioxidant, helping to form collagen (forget Botox!), build healthy bones and teeth, and heal wounds. Look for red berries, red and green bell peppers, green kiwi fruit, and juices from guava, grapefruit, and oranges.[5]

"To all my little Hulkamaniacs, say your prayers, take your vitamins, and you will never go wrong."[3]

—Hulk Hogan

A candy bar a day . . . ? You know what helps the most when you're feeling stressed—whether you're on deadline with an important project at work or your mother-in-law is just heading in for the weekend? The first things you turn to are a trusted friend and a good piece of chocolate. Now studies are showing that dark chocolate (not milk chocolate) lowers blood pressure and provides tons of great antioxidants for your system. But don't drink a glass of milk with it—the milk counteracts the positive effects of the chocolate when taken together.[6]

Signs You Might Need
to Find Yourself a Therapist

There are times when chatting with your friends about life's little hiccups is not cutting it anymore. You need an objective opinion—an expert who can help you sort through the messes in your life and give you a healthy perspective on what to focus on and what to chuck out the window. Here are some signs that you might need someone to lend a professional ear.

"Sleeping in" has gone extreme. If your friends have all been at work for hours by the time you roll out of bed in the morning, if you have forgotten what you look like with makeup on and your hair fixed, if your social life is dead and buried, then you might be depressed. Are you feeling sad—all the time? Do you feel worthless or guilty for no real reason? Have you lost your appetite, or are you having trouble concentrating or making the simplest decision? It might be time to figure out what's going on inside. The good news is, this dark blue phase is just a phase—you will come back into the light again.

You're screaming at the neighbor kids. If the feeling that you just can't take it anymore is rising in you with increasing regularity, you might need to get a grasp on your anger issues. Are you clenching your teeth and sweating from that increased heart rate? Are you resentful, irritated, and generally ready to throw a stiletto at every little inconvenience? Have you lost your sense of humor? Or have you even acted out—screaming, hitting, or verbally abusing someone? You can get control over these urges with a little help, so don't despair.

You just need some advice. Do you feel overwhelmed by a decision you're having to make? Are relentless questions looming over your head? You might benefit from just getting some objective advice from someone who's not tied into the situation. Sometimes it's great to have someone available who just has to listen to you talk for a while.

You hate your husband, boyfriend, other-important-relationship person. If you're fighting all the time, your relationship is probably not in a great place at the moment. In fact, you might not even care enough to fight anymore. Are you finding it really hard to trust him? Do you feel used, abused, or neglected? It might be time to have a good heart-to-heart with your guy. Having someone teach you how to disagree yet still communicate with love will be a great asset in your relationship. And you don't have to limit relationship counseling to romantic relationships—there are a lot of important people in your life, and if any of those relationships are feeling too stressed to move forward, consider getting an outside opinion.

You're starting to look less like America Ferrara and more like Victoria Beckham. Is your weight dropping dramatically? Are you exercising way more than you should and eating way less than you should? Are you obsessed with the pictures of Lindsay Lohan and Nicole Ritchie in the tabloids—in their seemingly perfect bodies? How often do you think about how you look? Have your friends or family said they're worried you have a problem? It might be time to listen to them and talk to someone who can help you get your diet and your body back on track. The journey away from an eating disorder is not easy, but good—no, great—things await those who dare to take th first step.

> "Do you know the only person who'd wanna listen to this? A mental health professional. And that's only because they get paid a hundred dollars an hour."
>
> —Jennifer Aniston as Rachel Green, *Friends* ™
> © Warner Bros. Entertainment Inc.

Quick
Beauty Secrets

Get a great haircut. Having a good hair day gives you confidence and has the power to actually make you happier. But if you're an on-the-go kind of girl, you'll need a haircut that is low maintenance. Book yourself some time at a nice salon, and shell out a little of that hard-earned cash to get a top-of-the-line cut. Ask the stylist to share his secrets for making you look salon-great every day.

Open up your face. Your eyes are the window to your soul, right? They're also the key to looking pretty! Even if you're running late and have to skip the eye shadow, take a second to curl your lashes and apply a quick coat of mascara. Brightening your eyes will open up your entire face! And use a dab of sheer gel blush—great because you don't have to use foundation first—and a bit of moisturizer to liven up your look. And if you have some downtime, remember to use an AHA (alpha hydroxy acid) to slough off those dead skin cells and apply some self-tanner for a sun-kissed glow.

It is better to be beautiful than to be good . . .
—Oscar Wilde

Luscious lips. Putting a little color on your lips can bring your whole look together or destroy it all with one fell swoop, so be strategic in your lipstick choices. Dark colors make your lips appear smaller. Lip liner should never be darker than your lipstick color. A glossy sheer color is great for summer; just make sure it's in your color range. And if you want to go for a fuller, more dramatic look, you can dab a bit of gloss in the center of your lower lip and you'll look Hollywood-ready![7]

Soft skin. No one wants to see your crusty heels or dried-out elbows, but did you know soft skin actually makes your personality, as well as your body, appear more supple and alluring? So put a bottle of lotion by the bed and lather down at night; you can even use nipple cream, designed for nursing moms, if your skin is really dry! Keep your feet sensuous—especially important during the summer sandal months—with skin-softening socks. You can order a pair online at the Avenue You Beauty Store, where it is always all about you! You can find the chic beauty warehouse online at **www.aveyou.com**. And if you enter promo code "FIVE" at checkout, you'll get a 15 percent discount on anything you purchase.

Pearly whites. Is your daily Starbucks run putting a strain on your beauty as well as your budget? If you drink a lot of tea or coffee, you're probably due for a teeth-whitening session. You can have this done professionally at your dentist, and even at some aestheticians' offices, or you can buy a kit to use at home.

Best Ways
to Become Healthier

> DWIGHT: Through simple concentration I can both raise
> and lower my cholesterol.
> PAM: Why would you raise your cholesterol?
> DWIGHT: So I can lower it.
>
> —from *The Office*

Look cool. Fortunately, giving up smoking, which increases women's heart disease risk two to four times and is the most preventable cause of premature death in the United States, is not only good for your health (you don't say!), but also good for your image nowadays. Gone are the days when smoking looked cool. It had its heyday when your great-grandmother Ava smoked long, thin cigarettes while sipping gin and tonic in her dressing gown and slippers, waiting for her hair to set on rollers. Fortunately, today a healthy, fit woman with glowing skin and a toned body is more admired than one with yellowed fingers and teeth and a raspy voice!

Move it! Thanks to all the wonders of modern-day technology—online shopping, e-mail, cell phones, remote controls—there is little if any reason to put aside our laptops and get up off the couch . . . except to get a snack. But the fact is that physically active women have a 60 to 70 percent lower risk of heart disease than inactive women. So aim for a total of thirty minutes of moderate-intensity exercise (such as brisk walking) every day. And it doesn't even have to be done all at once! How easy is that?

Lose it. Not mentally—physically! Easier said than done, but definitely worth the effort when you consider that being more than 30 percent over your ideal body weight makes you more likely to develop heart disease, even with no other risk factors. To figure out your customized healthy body weight (even if you're pregnant!) log on to www.dietitian.com/ibw/ibw.html for a healthy body calculator that helps you determine if you have a small or large frame and what your goal weight should be, and even provides a calorie chart for you to follow.

Don't stress. Studies show that your body's physiological reaction to high levels of sustained stress—increased blood pressure, outpouring of adrenaline, and other changes—makes you more susceptible to serious disorders such as heart disease. Depression, more often suffered by women, is also dangerous to the heart in both women and men. High blood pressure increases the heart's workload, weakening it over time. It also increases the risk of stroke, heart attack, kidney failure, and congestive heart failure. A blood pressure of under 140 systolic (top) and 90 diastolic (bottom), with 120/80 being optimal, should be aimed for.

Be fussy. The only way to lower your cholesterol is to be picky about what you will and won't eat. Women with total cholesterol over 200 are more susceptible to heart disease. The goal is to have an LDL ("bad" cholesterol) lower than 160 and HDL ("good" cholesterol) over 45, and to keep triglycerides, which are emerging as a significant predictor of risk in women, to 200 or even lower.[8] So save butter, cream, and ice cream for special occasions, and limit the amount of store-baked goods you eat for snacks on the go.

Things You Can Do
to De-Stress

When you find yourself ready to throw the dog out the window, eat a gallon of ice cream, spend $800 on a new tank top, or scream at the top of your lungs in the middle of your cubicle, it might be time to de-stress. Here are some ways you can calm yourself down before disaster strikes.

Prepare. Even though the last thing you want to think about at the end of a long, hard day at the office is all the stuff you have to do tomorrow, planning ahead will help you feel more in control and prepared. Do these two easy, practical things before you leave the office each day: Write down tasks in order of priority that need to be accomplished the next day. And take a few minutes to organize your desk so you can start the next day with a clear head.

Lists. It's completely annoying to get home from the grocery and realize you forgot one little—but very important—item from your list. So, in addition to a to-do list for work, keep shopping and errand lists up-to-date and with you at all times. It will help you avoid that constant nagging feeling that there are a million things you should be doing that you're not getting to.

Time out! No matter how much work you have to do, don't let yourself get stuck in a cycle of never-ending tasks. Turn off your cell phone and e-mail. Schedule some time to do nothing—watch all those TiVo'd episodes of *Grey's Anatomy* you have saved up. Browse a copy of *domino* magazine. Go to a long lunch. And under no circumstances should you feel guilty about "wasting" time this way. You're actually recharging your batteries to get a lot more work done down the road.

> "Stress is nothing more than a socially acceptable form of mental illness."[9]
>
> —Richard Carlson

Give in to temptations. If nothing else about your day is enjoyable, at least give your day a bit of a boost with a tasty treat. Grab a chocolate or cookies to enjoy for a few minutes with a cup of tea. Get a milkshake or dish up a bowl of ice cream to lift your spirits after dinner while watching TV and finishing off those last few e-mails. Of course, a healthy diet the majority of the time will help give you the energy and nutrients you need to cope and ward of illness, but what's wrong with an occasional treat to help get you through the day?

Exercise. Hang a punching bag up in your office. Take a quick jog around the block before dinner. Why? Fitness activities, especially aerobic-type exercises, are helpful in reducing anxiety. Some researchers have suggested that a chemical is released in the brain during aerobic exercise that helps the body mend itself from some of the harmful effects of stress. For this to be effective long term, however, you should exercise at least three days per week for at least thirty minutes each time.[10]

145

Secrets for Eating Out
When You're on a Diet

Research shows that the more you eat out, the more likely you are to be overweight.[11] But cooking three meals a day at home might not fit in well with your lifestyle—a girl needs to get out sometimes! So here are some tricks for ordering light from any menu—from wontons to chimichangas.

Mexican. Although Mexican food tends to be smothered in cheese and deep fried in oil, it is possible to celebrate Cinco de Mayo without tipping the scales afterward! Start with a cup of black bean soup or tortilla soup with light (or no) cheese. Then have chicken or shrimp fajitas or soft tacos made with whole wheat or corn tortillas. Skip the cheese, and have a little guacamole and lots of salsa. If you want a drink, skip the margarita. Most have more than three hundred calories of sugar and alcohol. Go with a light beer or tequila with lime juice and club soda instead.

Chinese. When you're craving some yummy takeout, you can still dish up some Chinese. Start with wonton, hot and sour, or egg drop soup. Skip the white or fried rice and ask for brown rice instead. Also, ask for your food to be prepared "dry wok" style when possible. Experiment with Chinese veggies, and opt for chicken, tofu, or seafood as your protein. And it's sad but true: you should avoid the sweet and sour sauce (full of sugar!), and be careful about the amount of nuts you eat if you're counting fat grams.

Japanese. Grab your friends and head to the sushi bar for a healthy dinner. Start with miso soup, edamame (soy beans), or salad. Skip the tempura dishes—fried is never good for you. Limit yourself to eight pieces of sushi wrapped in rice—that's two servings of starch. Watch higher-fat ingredients in rolls, such as cream cheese, avocado, and mayo in spicy tuna or crab; they add hundreds of calories. Sashimi is a great alternative.

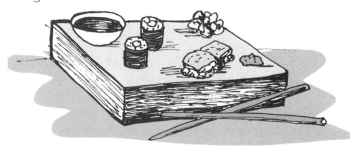

Delis. If the girls at the office are all going to the local deli for soup and sandwiches, you don't have to decline the invite. Just avoid mayo-based sandwiches, such as tuna salad, chicken salad, or egg salad, which contain hundreds of extra calories. Opt for lean meat and eat sandwiches open-faced. Order dressing on the side of any salad. Skip or remove most of the cheese and bacon on chef or cobb salads.

Steak house. Your guy's taking you out for a nice romantic dinner at the upscale steakhouse, but you don't have to worry about the hours you'll spend at the gym burning off your dinner. Start with a shrimp cocktail or salad (dressing on side), not the crab cakes. Opt for leaner cuts, such as filet mignon, instead of sirloin, prime rib, or porterhouse. Or even better, get their fresh catch! If you're craving a baked potato, eat half and limit the high-fat toppings. Stay away from the garlic mashed potatoes and creamed spinach, usually laden with cream.

Elements of a Truly Relaxing
At-Home Spa Night

The guest list. The most important factor in your relaxation is the people you invite to your spa night. This isn't the time to invite those people over who you've been avoiding for a few weeks and really should finally do something with, and it's not the time to invite the well-meaning but seriously depressing friend who will want to talk about her latest rash or boss problems. Invite only the friends you don't have to work hard to impress—the ones it's okay to be quiet around, whom you laugh easily with, and who will rejuvenate your spirit as you refresh your body.

Make it easy. The point is to be relaxing, right? So don't stress by spending hours researching the latest magazines and polling your local spas—unless you just really enjoy doing that kind of thing! Buy an at-home spa kit from **AveYou.com. If you enter "FIVE" at the checkout, you'll get a 15 percent discount on your purchase!**

Atmosphere. It's time to pull out the mood music or download some great songs from iTunes for your indulgent night. Some of our favorites are songs by Richard Hawley, Belle and Sebastian, Cat Power, Michael Bublé, John Lennon, Snow Patrol, Feist, Neil Young, and Corinne Bailey Rae.

Indulge. If you truly want to have a high-class, indulgent evening, consider hiring a masseuse or aesthetician to come do some pampering for your group. A masseuse can bring his own table, and you and your guests can take turns getting some deep-tissue relaxation. Sometimes there's just no equal to having a professional handle things!

Stock up. Be sure to have everything you'll need on hand—it's annoying to get halfway through a facial and realize you have no toner to finish it off! Have a stack of clean, warm towels, fresh bottles of all your beauty products, dim lighting, light but indulgent snacks, a pitcher of lemon water or ginger tea, and nice, fresh quilts for the girls to relax on.

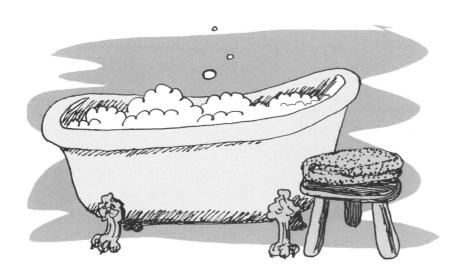

The Healthiest Foods
You Can Eat

There is a new diet on the market every day, and it's super-hard to know what is the right plan for you! Low carb? Low fat? All cabbage all the time? Yuck! So how do you weed through the dietary quagmire to figure out simple ways to eat healthy foods? Remember these basic tips from The World's Healthiest Foods.[12]

Nutrient dense. The brighter the color, the more nutrients the food has. And no, white is not a color!

Whole foods. This doesn't mean you should eat the "whole" pizza or the "whole" burrito! Instead, whole foods are basically foods in the same form they started out in. Have you ever seen a "Lean Cuisine" tree or a "hot dog" bush? Exactly—these boxed, processed, packaged, and highly marketed foods are not as good for you as fresh, wild-caught salmon or organic strawberries. Think of it this way: if it has a jingle, it's probably not on the healthiest list.

Familiar foods. Eat foods that you like, foods that you're comfortable with, and foods you know. You'll be less freaked out by changing your entire way of life—which some diets can do—and you'll remember to eat the things you should. Apples, bananas, chicken, beef—they're all good for you to eat! It's really not that hard, just stock up on healthy foods you already like to eat.

Readily available. You'll be more likely to eat healthily if you can get healthy foods easily. If you eat out a lot, find a restaurant you like with a great salad option or some lean grilled meats and fresh veggies on their menu. Shop at a grocery store with a good selection of produce that offers meats from animals whose diets consisted of whole grains and were given no hormones or antibiotics. And stick as much as possible to the perimeter of the grocery stores—the stuff on the aisles in the middle tends to be less healthy.

Junk food. Desserts and junk food aren't actually the healthiest thing you can eat—unless you consider a fresh fruit and yogurt smoothie a fantastic dessert. (We tend to go for Death by Chocolate Cake!) But cheating is important. If you tell yourself you can never have a sweet again because you're eating healthily now, you'll give up before long. So if you're at the ball game, grab a hot dog. If you're having a special night out at the theater, stop in for a fantastic crème brûlée afterward. Just don't do it every day, and your body will thank you!

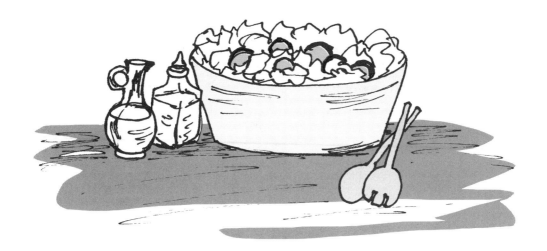

Questions to Ask Yourself
Before Starting a Diet

Why am I doing it? It is important to define your motivation for losing weight. Why do you really want to lose weight? To find a man? To fit into the jeans you wore in high school? To feel good about yourself? To be a role model for your children? For health concerns, current or future? If you're trying to please others rather than yourself, you'll probably be less likely to succeed.

Does it really matter if I'm overweight? Yes! Are you fully aware of the implications of being seriously overweight? Heart disease, arthritis, and diabetes are all potential side effects of obesity. Weight loss can help reduce your risk.

Is now a good time? What's coming up in your life in the next few months? Are you moving? Starting a new job? Taking an extended trip that you have been planning for two years? If you are making any major changes or have significant obligations in the next few months, it may not be the best time to start a diet. This time period is critical because it takes a month or two for new habits to become "second nature."

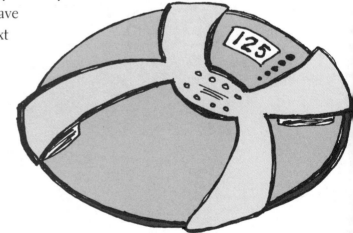

Will I ever look like Kate Moss? Are you hoping to get down to the weight you were in college, before the three kids, endless demands, and full-time job? What did it take to get and stay there back then? Not only has your lifestyle probably changed, but genetics and a slower metabolism could also make losing weight a little more difficult now. You may not be able to have the figure of a supermodel, but you can have a strong, fit, healthy body.

How fast can I lose it? Are you trying to drop twenty pounds before your trip to Cabo next month? Under most circumstances, you simply cannot lose weight that quickly, and if you do, you will probably lose a significant amount of muscle, water, and even bone. It is very difficult for women to lose more than one to two pounds of fat per week.[13]

Inside some of us is a thin person struggling to get out, but she can usually be sedated with a few pieces of chocolate cake.

—Author Unknown

Tips for Getting Through
Nine Months of Pregnancy Without Going Crazy

Those nine months when that precious new life is growing inside you is full of ups and downs. You've got that "pregnant glow." Or maybe it's just sweat glistening from those hot, sleepless nights. Flushed cheeks from days and days spent over the toilet bowl. And glistening eyes from the tears you've cried and cried, for no apparent reason except a violent shift in hormone levels! Here are some suggestions on surviving this hormonal ride of life.

The things to complain about. Morning sickness. Hemorrhoids. Heartburn. Cramping, stretching, and itching. What did I forget? I'm sure you've had some unique and strange ailment yourself—a sore tailbone or super-sensitive nipples! There are folk remedies and prescription medicines for most of these ailments. For some specific suggestions, log on to Childbirth.org.[14]

That awkward period where people aren't sure if you're pregnant or just fat. Even if you're not the type to advertise your new condition, this period may tempt you to find any excuse to tell *anyone* that you're expecting! "Yes, that's my car blocking the entrance. You know, gosh, I'm pregnant, and I just keep doing silly things like that!" If you're not the type to verbally explain your expanding waistline, check out the fun T-shirts at **2Chix.com**, which will do the talking for you. If you enter "Essential5" in the promo code box at checkout, you'll get a 10 percent discount on your purchase!

Unsolicited advice. It's sad but true—the unsolicited advice that starts during your pregnancy only gets worse after the baby comes. From comments on nursing, child safety, naming the baby, and more, it seems that everyone questions your right or ability to be a mother. Just ignore them and smile.

The nesting phase. This is easily the most expensive stage of pregnancy. If you're feeling the need to hide the receipts from your baby daddy, take a minute to breathe deep, calm down, and examine your current and future needs for the baby. A nursery is necessary, but a $1,500 crib might not be. Web sites will recommend hundreds of products as "must-haves" for your new bundle of joy, but take the time to talk to a friend with kids and find out what she actually uses day in and day out. You may find some great deals on brand-name items at consignment sales in your area too—check out KidsConsignmentSales.com for one near you.

Birth. The biggest piece of advice we can give on sailing through the birth process is to enjoy it. Try to soak it all in—except the contractions, the needles, and the countless people who will come in to look at your . . . progress. Be sure to look into your husband's eyes, relish the wonder of this new life coming from inside you, and see if you can't find a way to embrace the pain. No words can fully describe the moments of childbirth. It is truly an awe-inspiring and life-changing event in every way. Welcome that little child with all the love you've been building up for nine months and more!

Ways to Fight

Colds and the Flu

"Just what kind of flu have we have here, Doc?"

"That's an excellent question, Holling, that's an excellent question. A flu virus is named for its point of origin. Um, the Shanghai flu, the Hong Kong flu, the Russian flu, the Westchester . . ."

"So, it could be Russian flu?"

"Certainly."

"I never did trust Gorbachev."

—from *Northern Exposure*

Pick your battles. Many annoying cold symptoms are part of the natural healing process, so resist the urge to overmedicate yourself when your nose is running and your throat is itchy. Having a fever is the body's way of trying to kill viruses in a hotter-than-normal environment. Coughing clears your breathing passages of thick mucus that carries germs to the rest of your body. Even a stuffy nose is best treated mildly or not at all.[15]

Knock out fruit juices. You should load up on orange juice when you're feeling under the weather, right? Actually, no. Sugar impairs the immune system, and all fruit juices contain sugars. Instead, increase your intake of vitamin C *supplements* to 6,000 to 8,000 mg a day. Also, drink plenty of water, herbal tea, and vegetable juice to hydrate your respiratory tract.[16]

Take a shot. Most doctors recommend getting a flu shot—especially for the very young or very old, or those caring for either. Flu strains change year to year, and so do the vaccinations. You can get the flu shot at your doctor's office. Many health clinics, community centers, and even drugstores offer this yearly shot as well.

Have an arsenal. If your red and itchy eyes, runny nose, and incessant cough are interfering with your work or life to the point you can't stand it anymore, grab some over-the-counter medicine to temporarily manage the symptoms. You don't want to be sniffing like a toddler while your cutie boyfriend romances you or your boss is asking you to take over a new client.

The basics. If you're feeling like you've been run over by a truck, you should drink fluids, try to eat regularly, and get plenty of rest so that your body will have the energy it needs to attack the virus. Vitamin C is a powerful antioxidant that helps support the immune system in the battle against colds and flu, so try to fill up on citrus fruits, green leafy veggies, tomatoes, and capsicum. Also, garlic has antiviral and mucus-reducing properties which help the body's natural healing processes.

Exercises You Can Do
in Five Minutes

If your schedule rivals that of Ryan Seacrest during the Oscars and *American Idol* sweeps, you hardly have time for a two-hour "stiletto strength" class at the gym. Instead, do each of these exercises for one minute. Try to do them at least three times a day—and look for creative opportunities to fit them in. Making copies at the office? Do some calf strengtheners. Playing on the floor with the kids? Let them crawl under your bridge pose.

Bridge pose. Lay on the floor on your back with your hands at your sides. Pull your shoulder blades down and relax your core—be sure your back is flat on the ground. With your feet shoulder-width apart, lift your hips straight up in the air as high as is comfortable for you. (Don't raise them beyond your comfortable "edge" or you'll strain your back.) Bring your hands together on the floor and clasp them together. Take deep breaths as you count to sixty. Release!

Calf strengtheners. Stand very straight—head over shoulders, shoulders over hips, hips over knees. Keep your feet shoulder-width apart as you raise your body up on the balls of your feet, then lower with your heels just hovering over the floor. Do this for thirty seconds. Now move your feet closer together—balls of your feet touching, heels just slightly apart. Raise and lower for thirty more seconds.

Arm toners. Grab two cans of soup or two bottles of water and work out those arm muscles. With a can in each hand, hold your arms out straight in front of you, palms facing down. Slowly lower your arms to your thighs then back up to shoulder-height. Repeat this ten times. Then, move your arms out to your sides as if forming a T with your body, and repeat ten more times. Finally, drop your hands to your hips, palms facing upward (still holding the cans/bottles), and curl them up toward your shoulders. Repeat this ten times!

Downward-facing dog. This simple yoga pose provides a real workout when held for a good long stretch. Start with your hands and knees on the floor. Turn your toes under and lift with your hips so that your body forms a V shape toward the ground. Your head and neck should be in line with your arms, and your arms and legs should be soft yet straight. Put the weight of your body back into your heels, and hold for sixty seconds.

Walk around. Take the long route to the coffee station at work, walk in place during a commercial break, or park far from the door when you go to the mall. Keep your body moving and your heart rate going! Really pick your knees up as you go, as if you were marching. Keep your arms pumping while you walk. If you have kids at home, they will love playing with you on this one!

Ways to Stay
Motivated at the Gym

That first week back at the gym is often pure bliss, tempered only by that slight soreness that reminds you how good it feels to be working out again! But beware—around week two or three your energy will drain, excuses will rise, and you will find yourself struggling to stay motivated. Here are some strategies to stay in the game.

Have a goal outfit. There is *some* reason you're motivated to lose weight—an upcoming event, bathing-suit season approaching, or jealous that the models in J. Crew magazines are so darn good looking. Your trick? Buy an outfit you wish you could wear in the size you're aiming to be, and hang it up where you can see it every day. Let it be your inspiration to shed a few pounds.

Get out the digital camera. For the truly daring, a good motivator is the brutal truth. Take some photos of yourself in the buff, print them on your home photo printer (please don't use the color copier at work!), and hang one on your bathroom mirror. If you're not quite that sure of yourself—or if you have frequent visitors to your bathroom—take one in a bikini or a favorite outfit that has gotten too small.

Find an exercise partner. It's a lot easier to stay dedicated when you know someone else is counting on you to show up. Pick a friend who's not afraid to tell it like it is and will let you have it if you bail on her. Find a time that works for both of you, and meet up to exercise. Take a walk in the park if you're the talkative type. Join a kickboxing class if you're the high-impact type.

Be lazy. It's important to cheat once in a while when you're putting yourself through such an emotional ringer as diet and exercise lifestyle changes. If you give yourself infrequent indulgences, you'll be more likely to stay the course over the long haul.

Have a tangible goal. Make a real, measurable goal for yourself for the near future. For example, *I want to lose five pounds by next month.* Every time you meet the goal, set a new one. Also, make some intangible goals for yourself. *I want to make my ex completely regret dumping me when I see him at the wedding next summer. I want my mom, for once, not to mention shedding a couple of pounds when she visits me.*

Never eat more than you can lift.

—Miss Piggy

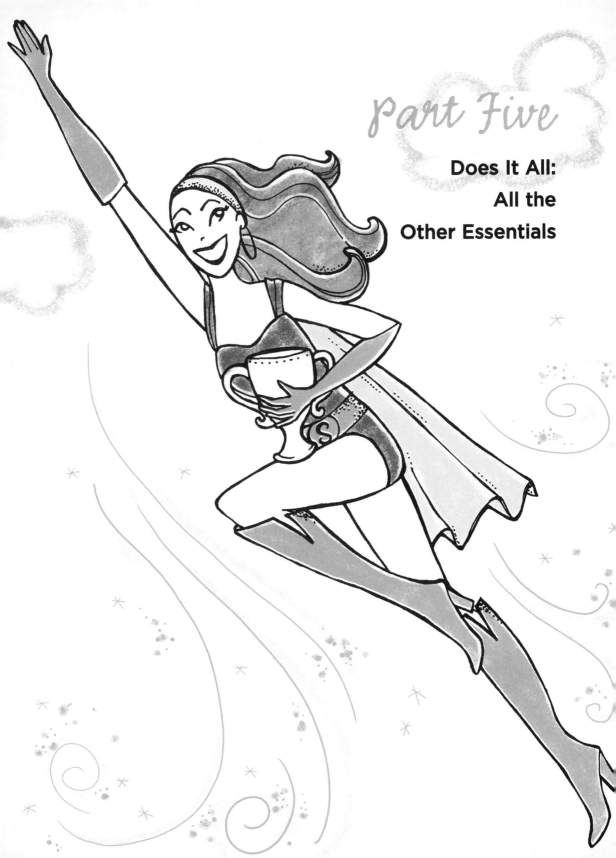

Part Five

**Does It All:
All the
Other Essentials**

Games Every Woman
Should Know How to Play

"Are you sure you guys want to play for money?
Phoebe just threw away a pair of jacks because they didn't look
   happy."

> —David Schwimmer as Ross
> on "The One with the Poker," *Friends* ™
> © Warner Bros. Entertainment Inc.

Poker. Poker tournaments are all over the TV lately; in fact, you can probably see a card game any time of the day. It's crossing over from TV to our social lives too. You need to know to hold your own in a game of Texas Hold'em, the most popular of the poker games at the moment. It'll impress the guys—and perhaps even make you a couple of bucks along the way. Visit the World Poker Tour Web site (www.worldpokertour.com) for rules and strategies.

Hard to get. Most every guy has something programmed in him that makes him want to win, to get the prize, to return victorious. So indulge him a little by playing hard to get. Now, I'm not saying you should be an ice princess—this is not an exercise in the cold shoulder. What will drive him crazy, in a good way, is the subtle ways you'll keep him wondering, make him curious to know what makes you tick, and whet his appetite to discover more.

164

Golf. It may seem boring; it can certainly be boring to watch on TV. But golf is—despite the cliché—a game you can play the rest of your life. It's also a game that can get you some one-on-one time with your CEO, endear you to your future father-in-law, or give you an excuse to spend four hours away from the chores of home and out with your girlfriends in the warm sunshine! Take a lesson, buy some cute gear, and get out there and play. The benefits are great, and you may find out it's not so boring after all.

Dumb. We've come a long way, girls, in the fight for equality. We all know women are intelligent, capable, self-reliant human beings who can make a difference in this world as well as any man can. But we have one secret weapon men can't get away with—playing dumb. We can use it to let people—ourselves or others—off the hook, to get out of a traffic ticket, and to avoid chastisement from just about anyone. By playing dumb in the "I'm really very willing to learn how to avoid this mistake again" vein, you might be able to go places you didn't expect.

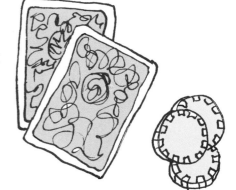

Video games. You probably grew up in the video-game generation. Those of us who were raised on Atari and Nintendo have fond memories of Super Mario Brothers, Pac Man, and Q-Bert. But video games are here to stay—for better or worse. If you're a total novice, and your boyfriend loves to play, find a game that is fun for you too. Try party games like Dance, Dance Revolution, Mario Party, or Wii Play games. Or, if you have kids at home who like gaming, you should be aware of what's in the games they're playing. Most include some level of violence and bad language, but you'll definitely want to keep an eye out for anything rated M (for mature)—they can include nudity and *excessive* violence, and they're usually more "mature" than R-rated films.

Words You Should Say
If You Want to Sound Smart

PETER: Brian, there's a message in my Alphabits. It says, "Oooooo."
BRIAN: Peter, those are Cheerios.

—from *Family Guy*

Small words. We've all come across people who try to make themselves sound smarter by using big words that no one else understands. According to a study by Princeton psychologist Daniel Oppenheimer, people can see through this. In his study he used a thesaurus to replace the simple words in writing samples with needlessly flowery ones and gave both copies to students to evaluate. The result? "As the grandiosity and complexity of the language increased, the judges' estimation of the author's intelligence decreased."[1]

I. Believe it or not, most people don't know how to talk about themselves properly! "Myself" is an often incorrectly used—and overused—word in our society. And ironically, "myself" is often used in an attempt to sound *more* intelligent. For example, most people would say: "Maria, Linda, and myself went to work," when you should say, "Maria, Linda, and I went to work."[2] Quick tip: think of how you would say the sentence if the other names weren't in there—would you ever say, "Myself went to work"?

That, who, or which. Do you find yourself getting flustered trying to decide which one of these words to use and end up resorting to "that" all the time? Here's a quick tip for remembering: "that" applies to things, "who" applies to people, and "which" applies to information that could be left out of a sentence. For example, "The gift *that* he bought for you is amazing!" "The woman *who* just got out of the car is beautiful," and "When I finish work, I'm going to watch *Jerry Maguire, which* is a real tearjerker."[3]

Improving your vocabulary. The best way to truly improve your vocabulary, and not sound like you've swallowed a thesaurus is to read a lot and look up the words you don't know. You can do the same when watching TV. The more language you're exposed to, the more new words you'll learn. Try to make it a habit to add a new word in your vocabulary each week! For book suggestions, turn to "Ways to Pick a Book You're Sure to Love" on pages 72-3, or tune in to *The Daily Show* or *The Colbert Report* to pick up some impressive—but not too impressive—words.

Zip it! Sometimes the most intelligent thing to do is to shut up. This is described perfectly in the proverb "Even a fool is thought wise if he keeps silent, and discerning if he holds his tongue."[4] So, when you don't really have anything to contribute but feel compelled to speak up to look smart, *zip it* (as Dr. Evil would say in the Austin Powers movies). Holding your tongue can be a sure way to fool people into thinking you're smarter than you really are!

Annual Appointments
to Make—and Keep!

Your life is crazy busy, and it's positively annoying to have to take vacation time off of work or hire a babysitter just to go to the doctor. But there are some annual appointments you really do need to keep. As the old saying goes, "An ounce of prevention is worth a pound of cure."

Medical. We hate it, but we need to do it. Pick a time of year that will help you remember to visit the doctor—whether it's your birthday, the new year, or some other significant date that reminds you just a bit of your mortality. Visit your general practitioner for a full checkup and go see your ob-gyn to make sure everything's working smoothly down there as well.

Financial analyst. It's a good idea to check in regularly on your finances. Make an appointment around tax time with an analyst who can help you reevaluate your goals and visualize your progress toward them.

Home maintenance. It's easy to forget the simple things you have to do to keep your home running smoothly, but it's much more frustrating to buy a new air conditioner than it is to get new filters. Mark your calendars to replace your air filters regularly, have your heating and air-conditioning units checked twice a year, get your carpets deep cleaned, and keep up with all household maintenance. And hire a maid to come in and do all the gross work you just don't feel like doing!

Personal care. Take a day to treat yourself—skip work, get a massage or pedicure, take a leisurely lunch at your favorite restaurant, and get in bed early with your favorite movie (or your cute hubby!). Make it a day about you. It'll revive you for spending your time giving to others in your "real" life.

Soul care. If you're not a regular at confession or do not see a counselor, take one day a year to get it all out. Schedule it near the Lenten season or Yom Kippur. If you have emotional baggage you've been carrying around, get rid of it! You'll be amazed at the freedom you'll find in letting go of the past.

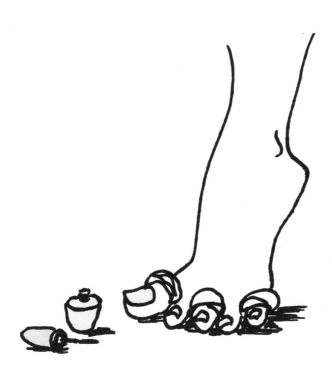

Things You Need to Know
So You Don't Get Hosed by a Mechanic

When you get your car serviced or repaired, you have two options: the vehicle dealership or an independent shop. The choice, as always, involves a trade-off: independent shops are usually cheaper, but dealerships have more accountability and a dealer warranty. But, the truth is, no matter which one you choose, you run the risk of falling prey to time-honored tricks. Here are some great tips from ServiceSnitch.com on what you need to know when dealing with auto mechanics, and what you have to do to protect yourself from getting hosed.

Choosing a mechanic. When considering a repair shop—and you should consider several before deciding on one—ask for references. You should also ask the mechanics whether they have certification from the National Institute for Automotive Service Excellence (ASE). No matter how many certificates or awards a shop has, however, always call your local Better Business Bureau to see if any complaints have been filed against them. Finally, ask the shop if they guarantee their service; if so, have them put it in writing.

Ask for an estimate. Always ask for an estimate with a detailed explanation before any repairs are made and before you commit to anything! Are all the parts and accessories covered? Do they anticipate you'll have to pay for something else? As always, once you have an estimate, shop around. If a garage tells you they can't make any estimate before beginning work on the car, wait until you hear a few more opinions.

Unexpected problem with a relatively new car. If you have an unexpected problem with a relatively new car, check the National Highway Traffic Safety Administration's Web site and search for your make and model to find any recalls or technical service bulletins (TSBs). A "recall" is a defect acknowledged by the manufacturer, while a TSB is a defect that enough people have noticed to merit attention. If the problem with your car is listed, you can usually get your car serviced at the dealership free of charge.

Scheduled maintenance. Before taking your vehicle for scheduled maintenance, check the owner's manual to see what parts need to be serviced or replaced at that time. If the mechanic insists that your car needs more service than what the manual suggests, show him your research and see what he says. Chances are he'll back off his initial assessment pretty quickly!

Repair. If you're taking your car in for repair, buy a service manual (also called a "repair manual" or "shop manual") for your model. It tells you, on average, how much time all sorts of different repairs take. It is what mechanics use to estimate their prices. Read up on the service you need. That way, when you take your car to the garage, you'll know what the mechanic is 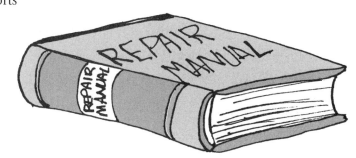 talking about and he won't be able to fast-talk you into an inflated invoice. You can find a manual at automotive specialty outfits such as Pep Boys and AutoZone.[5]

Ways to Stay
In-the-Know

Befriend a blabbermouth. Is there that one person in your social circle who knows everything about everybody? Give her a call now and again to stay current on the need-to-knows in your social world. But beware what you say; anything you tell her will be public knowledge as soon as you hang up the phone.

Hang out by the watercooler. Skip the meetings, delete the mass e-mails, but do not—I repeat, *do not*—quit hanging out by the watercooler. All important information you need to know at your company, you'll find out there. Layoffs coming up? New executive promotion available in your department? Another reorganization and new cubicle assignments? These topics will all be covered, and usually the one in the know is the assistant to the big guy.

Call your mom. Stay in touch with your mom, and you'll stay current on all the family drama—as well as find out key info on old high school friends and other locals from your past. Ask her what she's heard lately at church or at the grocery store. She'll love giving you the dish on all her—and your—old friends.

Reset your home page. Set your home page on your Internet browser to the BBC (news.bbc.co.uk) or some other news organization. Even if you don't read the articles, you'll see the headlines when your screen pops up eac morning. So when your boss surprises you by asking you to come along to lunch, you'll be able to ask, "So what do you think about . . . ?" and you'll sound really up-to-date!

Multitask in the checkout line. While you're waiting in the grocery store checkout line, browse the headlines on all the gossip magazines. You can get up-to-date on all things pop culture without having to waste precious time and energy actually reading articles about Justin Timberlake's new romance or Scarlett Johansson's latest hairstyle.

I can always keep a secret.
It's the person I tell it to who can't.
—Author Unknown

Ways to Get Rid of Pests
(from Cockroaches to Your Mother-in-Law)

We've all had the unwanted guest at our home—whether it's a family of ants taking over your kitchen or a Dupree-like friend who just won't leave. Here are some ideas for kicking out those unwelcome visitors while still keeping on good terms with those you want to!

Don't invite them in the first place. All pests are attracted to your home by something specific—mice like the warm environment, ants like crumbs, and your boyfriend's annoying friends like your big-screen TV. So figure out a way to make sure the pest in your life understands he is not invited to share your living space with you—whether you have to do a deep clean on the kitchen or plan an all-night *Gilmore Girls* marathon.

Be a bad host. If the pesky intruder has, in fact, found a way into your home, do your best to make your house inhospitable. Remove any creature comforts the pest may crave. Hide the poker chips and rid the fridge of beer. Scour the kitchen floor with vinegar and water. If you've got guests you don't want to be rude to—such as parents or in-laws visiting from out of town—but you feel like it's time for them to head on home, let them know your schedule is going to fill back up pretty soon. Inform them that you will be going back to work—which will at least give you a break from their constant attention.

Bait them. If steps one and two have failed, it's time to bait your pest. Pull out the sticky strips and mousetraps. Grab the peanut butter and cheese. Use their longings against them. Is your annoying book club buddy lingering too long after the discussion has ended? Figure out what she is looking for (someone to talk to), give her an appealing alternative (recommend that great literature chat room you just visited), and send her on her way!

Trap them. Sometimes pesticide is your only alternative. The sound of a mousetrap snapping shut is both chilling and strangely fulfilling. For the creatures that have overtaken your home, you can buy poison at the hardware or grocery store. Or you can call in the experts for larger furry pests. When you're dealing with a human intruder, you have to be clever. Make them think the decision to leave is their own. If your control-freak mother-in-law has "been so kind as to bring dinner over" twice this week already, let her know you're going to be massively overworked in a couple of weeks and could really use her help then.

Be humane. The ultimate rule to remember is be kind in releasing pests back into the wild. Whether you've hired a humane animal trapper who takes the squirrels running through your walls back to his friendly farm in the countryside or you're finally getting up the guts to tell your parents you can't take it anymore and they have to leave *now*, do it with gentleness and compassion. No one wants to be unwanted.

Things to Do
When You're So Mad, You Can't See Straight

We all know how it feels to be blind with rage after being falsely accused at work or shunned by a loved one. Here are some much-needed tips to keep in mind the next time you get so mad you are tempted to throw logic and caution to the wind!

The sanity gap. Most people cannot think straight, never mind see straight, when they're "blind with rage." In these cases the wisest thing to do is to take a time-out until you can think logically again. You don't want to do or say something you will regret later! Do whatever you can to resist the powerful urge to retaliate, whether face-to-face, over the telephone, or via e-mail. Give yourself at least twenty-four hours until you can think straight again.

Vent! The best way to occupy your time during the seemingly unbearable sanity gap is to let off steam in a safe environment. Let someone you trust know how you think and feel. But make sure your confidante isn't going to get so worked up on your behalf that she'll want to rush to your defense to make the situation right.

Distraction. For the remainder of the twenty-four-hour sanity gap, counteract the way you are going to feel until the issue is resolved by doing something that will distract you from your anger. Grab a coffee and sweet treat with a friend, watch a movie, go shopping—whatever you do should make yourself feel better. Don't sit at home alone and stew!

Plan your response. Once the twenty-four-hour time-out is over, sit down and plan your response to whatever it was that made you so mad. You'll be able to think a lot clearer now, as well as with a bit of hindsight and logic. And knowing how you will react will take the emotional irrationality out of your backlash.

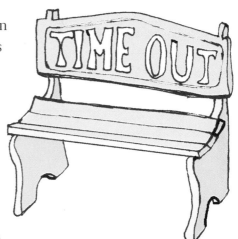

Get good counsel. Before you carry out your response, go over your plan with someone you view as wise counsel. Of course, you know the situation best and have to make the final decision about what you do, but take the advice from your counsel into account. You may be surprised what an objective mind might notice or come up with that you could have missed.

Things You
Should Fake

No one is perfect at everything, and there comes a time when we all need to fake our way through the tough spots. So when is it okay to pretend you're something you're not?

Your capabilities. You're at a big meeting with a new client when he pops the question, "Can you do. . . ?" You've never done it before, but you're sure you can figure it out or find someone to do it for you. "Yes!" you confidently answer. Or maybe your cute new date wants to go hiking—*hiking*? You *love* hiking, right? Just scramble to borrow some boots from a friend and suggest a leisurely trail so the two of you can chat while you walk, er, hike.

Your sense of style. You know stylish when you see it, and you know it when you don't. But you're afraid your home-wardrobe-hair is desperately falling short, and you're not sure what to do about it. Grab a copy of *domino* magazine or schedule some time to watch HGTV to get specific ideas for your apartment; hire a personal shopper to help you pick out some new clothes; find a fab hairstylist and completely trust him or her with your hair makeover.

Your culinary skills. You can't cook scrambled eggs, much less a meal for the dinner party for twelve you're hosting next weekend. Don't sweat—your friends and family will think you're the next Giada De Laurentiis, and there's no reason for them to know better! Stop by your favorite restaurant or deli on your way home. Simply transition the takeout from the plastic containers onto your trendy serving dishes, and voila! You're a gourmet chef!

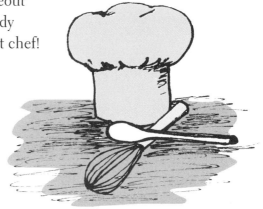

Your satisfaction. You know the look that crosses your face when you open a gift and it's a set of crocheted potholders, not a cashmere wrap from Barney's. Or the look you make when your mother-in-law says she just booked a week's vacation for the whole family—in a *cozy* 400-square-foot cabin in the woods? Or the one when your boss asks you to go on that last-minute sales trip to Wichita over the weekend, and you were supposed to be going to Miami with your friends? Take some time to stand in front of the mirror and practice a genuine-looking fake smile, a thank-you that will pass for sincere, or a "Sure, I'd be glad to" that sounds convincing.

Well, you know . . . Life gets pretty busy sometimes, and it's hard to find time for romance between the bills, the kids, and *CSI*. But even if you aren't in the mood, you do feel it's important to do the deed with some regularity. So, if you're not feeling it, fake it. Pretending you're having a great time doing anything—even sex—can be a great mind teaser. Who knows, maybe it won't end up being so fake after all!

Ways You Can
Save the World

You're probably thinking, *Wow! Save the world? What about finding time to fix the blocked garbage disposal?* You're right. Home comes first, and you probably have a list a mile high to see to. But doing a small part to help fix the world, your city, and your neighborhood doesn't have to be as time-consuming as it sounds.

Start at home. Green is the new black—being environmentally conscious is the newest hip thing. And there are tons of ways to get involved without having to miss *The OC* reruns. Conserve water by installing a toilet dam; it cuts down on water each time you flush. Save energy by putting in a programmable thermostat—does your house really need to be a cool 68 degrees when you're at the office? For more ideas, check out EarthShare.com.

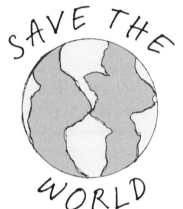

Superwoman! You're on board; you're inspired; you're ready to make a difference in a big way. But where do you start? Pick three charities you want to get involved with—one local, one national, and one international. With a little research you can easily find a convenient way to assist those in need in your city, your country, and the world as a whole!

Love your neighbors. There are many needs that go unnoticed, and often they are the unknown needs of neighbors you see every day. The elderly, the lock-and-key children, and the single mothers, for instance. By taking the time to look out for these invisible needs, and then offer a helping hand, you will be taking a big step toward making the world a place where love, not selfishness, and giving, not busyness, actually exist.

Be vocal. One of the easiest ways to make a difference is to let someone else do the work for you. Do you realize you have a whole staff of people fighting for the issues you think are important—your representatives in government. So get online and write a letter to your senator (it's super easy) about anything you want to see changed in the world. And stay on him to make sure he votes the way you want him to! All you have to do is go to www.congress.org and enter your zip code, and all your representatives will pop up with links for you to e-mail them.

Do nothing! We all know one of "them," and if you don't, it might be you! We're talking about those busybodies who seem to have too much time on their hands; all they do is look for something to complain about. They're the ones who patrol the neighborhood on a regular basis and complain unnecessarily about petty issues at the homeowners' association meetings. They tell the boss you were at lunch five minutes too long today. Instead of making the community a better place, these nosy neighbors only create work for everyone else. It would be better for everyone if they would just "do nothing!"

Steps
of CPR

In an emergency, knowing CPR can be the difference between life and death. Take the time to sign up for a class at the Red Cross to be fully trained in the procedure, but read through these steps to have some know-how in the meantime.

Check for unresponsiveness. Sometimes a person in cardiac arrest may make grunting, gasping, or snoring sounds for a couple of minutes. Do not be confused by this abnormal type of breathing. If a person is unresponsive (doesn't respond to shouts or shakes) and is not breathing (or is breathing abnormally) then CPR is needed.

Call. If the victim is unresponsive, call 911 from her side. If the victim is a child and you are alone, give two minutes of CPR before calling 911. In most locations the emergency dispatcher can assist you with CPR instructions. Also, if you're alone, shout for help—a neighbor or passerby may hear you and come to help you assist the victim. But don't panic, you need to keep your focus to help your friend in need.

Blow. Tilt the person's head back and listen for breathing. If the victim is not breathing *normally*, pinch his nose, cover his mouth with yours, and blow until you see the chest rise. Give two breaths. Each breath should take two seconds.

Pump. If the victim is still not breathing normally, coughing, or moving, begin chest compressions. Interlace your fingers with your hands one on top of the other (that is, the palm of one hand against the back of the other hand). Press the chest down one and a half to two inches thirty times, right between the nipples. Pump at the rate of one hundred times per minute, faster than once per second. You may hear a cracking sound. Do not be alarmed. The sound is caused by cartilage or ribs cracking—not serious damage compared to the risk of not performing CPR. (If you're doing CPR on a child, use the heel of one hand, and press the sternum approximately one-third the depth of the chest.)[6]

Focus. When you have a friend or loved one suffering from a heart attack, his only chance of survival is to get his heart beating again. You must stay focused. Keep your own breathing steady and focus on the task at hand—do not panic or lose your calm. If you can keep it together, you may be able to save the life of this person you love.

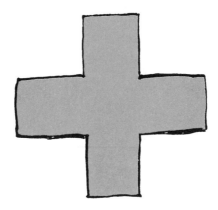

Tips for a
Successful Career

If we have to work, we might as well be successful, right? Nationally known career and job expert Randall S. Hansen, PhD, is the founder of one of the oldest and most comprehensive career development sites on the Web, Quintessential Careers (www.quintcareers.com). Here's his expert advice on how you can climb to the top of that corporate ladder.

Don't worry, be happy. No matter your age or your current employment situation, if you are unhappy with the type of job you perform, it's eventually going to have a bad effect on all aspects of your life. Take a weekend—or a couple of them—and complete some self-reflection on what you really want to do with your life. Once you discover your career passion, develop a plan for achieving it. Make sure you also research the corporate cultures of the organizations where you want to work to make sure they fit with your values.

No workaholics allowed. There's a difference between being ambitious and hardworking, and simply overdoing it. Your life—and your career—will be so much better if you can carve out a balance (that fits you) between work and home. While certain employers and careers are much more balance friendly, almost all employers recognize the value of retaining happy and healthy employees. And if full-time employment is no longer an option, consider job sharing or telecommuting.

What women do best. The most powerful tool in job hunting should come easy to most women—making friends and building relationships, otherwise known as networking. People with whom you have some kind of relationship are in your network, including family, friends, coworkers, associates, bosses, and the like. Keep expanding your network, and keep up with your current network, and new career opportunities will find you. You should belong to at least two professional organizations and two social organizations—and not just belong, but participate (and build those relationships).

The mysterious salary gap. Why is the gap between salaries for men and women so wide? One theory suggests that men enjoy the art of salary negotiation much more than women, who tend to accept an employer's first offer. The trick to salary negotiation is research—knowing what you are worth in the market and what the employer is willing to pay. And remember that almost all elements of a job offer are negotiable—not just the salary.

Market yourself. You probably know this already, but the best candidates are not always the ones selected for a new job or a promotion. The women who get ahead are the ones who track their accomplishments and make sure their bosses are aware of them—either through informal discussions or during annual reviews. Become an expert by writing articles in your field and serving as a spokesperson in the media.

Things You Need to Know
about Sports to Be One of the Boys

Shut up. While your guy may want you to be interested in sports, he doesn't want you asking incessant questions during the big game. If you're interested in learning, do it between tip-offs. And definitely do not try to have that serious heart-to-heart talk (even if it's about him spending too much time watching games and not enough time with you) during the game—you waited this long, now wait till the game is over.

Take what you can get. If your guy asks you to watch the game with him, that may be his weird way of asking you to spend time with him—even if he doesn't pay much attention to you. So cozy up with him and grab your favorite magazine to keep you entertained, then make him go with you to the mall to look for shoes later.

Don't be an expert. Guys, as a rule, are not looking for girls to be their sports trivia buddies—they have other guys for that. You're not going to win him over by memorizing RBI stats as much as you would by being a charming, considerate, fun date. So, if sports aren't your thing, don't force it. Be interested, but don't be a poser.

Find an entry point. If you're ready to learn a little bit about sports, but you don't really understand what's going on in the game, find an entry point that gets you excited. *Sports Illustrated* magazine publishes a great article by Rick Reilly on the very back page of every issue. It's always a compelling human interest

186

story about the sports world. Grab your guy's copy and read it. You'll surprise him with bits of info he won't expect you to know!

His fantasy. Indulge him and let him live out his fantasy. Fantasy football, baseball, basketball, or whatever that is. One guy tells us, "Fantasy sports are a strange and wonderful world. If your guy is into it and you don't get it, don't try to understand." Just let him have his fun—and cheer him on as he wins in his league week to week!

"Men forget everything.
Women remember everything.
That's why men need
instant replay in sports.
They've already forgotten
what happened."

—Rita Rudner

Things You Should

Always Have in Your Car

You may never leave home without your lipstick, cell phone, and breath mints. But have you taken the time to make sure you're fully prepared in case of an emergency in your car? Emergencies do happen, and having these things on hand could make all the difference!

Information. You probably never moved the owner's manual out of the glove compartment after you bought your car, but have you ever looked through it? It most likely has instructions on how to handle a variety of roadside disasters, such as how to change a flat tire. Get in the habit of throwing all the receipts from regular maintenance in there too. Keep a copy of your auto insurance policy, your AAA membership number, and a map of the state you're in with you as well.

Communication. Just in case you end up in an emergency without your cell phone, it is always a good idea to have an old one, even without a service plan on it, in the car. It can be powered on to call 911 or 999. Also, if weather conditions are atrocious, a battery-powered radio and extra batteries (or, even better, a crank-powered radio so you don't have to worry about batteries) can get you in touch with someone if you need help.

First-aid kit. Time to go shopping! Find a cute bag or box and keep it stashed full of first-aid items you might need. Emergency ice packs, ace bandages, a wrist brace, sunscreen, tweezers, straight-edge razor blades, wet wipes, safety pins, various OTC medicines (such as Tylenol and Benadryl), and tourniquets. Having something to slow bleeding could be the difference between life and death, and having an extra safety pin is very convenient if you break a strap on your dress when you're out at a party!

Survival kit. In addition to your first-aid kit, you'll need some survival items in the trunk as well—especially if you get stranded somewhere in the dark, in the cold, alone and miserable. A comfy blanket, fresh bottles of water, energy bars. An extra change of clothes, towels (to dry off with or put under a tire for traction), and cold-weather accessories, such as a cute hat and scarf set. Who says style has to suffer just because you're stranded? And throw in a magazine or book for good measure—it'll give you something to do while you wait for your knight in shining armor to come save you.

The standard stuff. Maybe you're not ready to channel your memories of Y2K preparedness quite yet, but you still have some essential items you really need to keep in your car. Jumper cables, spare tire, a jack, flares, a flashlight (and extra batteries), WD-40, a fire extinguisher, and portable battery charger will all come in very handy should you get stuck. If you are especially handy, keep a tool-box in the trunk too.[7]

Ways to Spend Less
at the Grocery

No matter what you plan to buy when you go to the grocery, it always seems that the total is way more than you expected. Do you graze the aisles while you shop—*ooh, that looks yummy! Oh, I heard that's super-healthy!* Here are some tried-and-true ideas to help you keep to your budget when shopping for food.

Make a list. Making a list and sticking to it is the best way to keep the total low when you go to the grocery. But be thorough when you're creating your list—that way you won't be able to make excuses when you "remember" that you really needed to get a new bottle of perfume and a copy of *Us Weekly* too. Planning your meals for the week goes hand in hand with this principle— knowing what you're going to cook eliminates impulse buying and overbuying.

Clip coupons. Don't be embarrassed to save money. Get the Sunday paper and clip coupons for the items you use regularly, but don't start buying tons of new stuff just because you have a coupon. And use your store's discount or VIP program—you can save an average of 10 to 15 percent doing these two things.

Eat. Don't go to the store hungry. You run the risk of being tempted to buy foods not on your list. Eat before you go, and you'll keep the total low.

Pay cash. If you set a budget for yourself at the beginning of the week and pay only with cash at the grocery, you'll be less likely to overspend on impulse purchases when you get there. You know before you go how much you will spend.

Don't join a cost-saving club. The idea of joining one of those huge warehouse price-slashing clubs for your grocery purchases sounds great, but in reality you can end up spending a lot more than you need to unless you have a big family to feed. The prices may be good for the amount you're getting, but do you really need two gallons of peanut butter this week?

Tips for Giving
a Seal-the-Deal Presentation

If the idea of giving a presentation has your knees knocking, here are some tips for making it a killer show that will bring in the big bucks for your business.

Don't overdo the graphics. Use visual aids in your presentation, but keep the PowerPoint limited. You don't want the audience reading your whole speech—you want them listening to your every word! So enhance the main points only in your visuals, use art sparingly, and focus on maximizing the effect of the *details* you want to communicate in your visuals.

Exude confidence. You want your audience to admire, respect, and look up to you. Wear your best clothes. Style your hair beforehand, but don't play with it when you're there! Fidgeting or fooling with your appearance detracts from your overall package, and that's what you're ultimately selling—yourself.

Be prepared. Know your topic back and forth. Don't *rely* on notes to speak (it's okay to have them as an outline), but talk straight from your knowledge of the subject. Know it well enough to answer any question your audience may ask. Know it well enough that you won't be caught off guard or distracted by tangent discussions or unavoidable mishaps—such as the fire alarm going off or people creeping in late. Your expert knowledge will win them over.

Fake it. If you aren't sure of the answer to a question you are asked, fake it. If you know enough about it to make a split-second decision, do that. So, *are you able to provide valet parking for all attendants to this conference you're planning?* Well, you hadn't thought of that, but *yes—no problem.* If you aren't able to decide right then and there, honestly and without your nerves coming undone, say you'll plan to look into that and get back to them in twenty-four hours. *That's a great idea we haven't discussed yet. We'll run the figures and get back to you tomorrow.*

Claim your territory. By staking your claim to the physical space where the presentation is being made, you'll make an impression beyond what your speech and graphics can convey. If you're pitching a board of sixty-something men at a publishing company with a book idea for teenage girls, cover the boardroom table with teen magazines, glitter nail polish, and funky fashion accessories. Creating an environment that matches your goals will give otherwise uninitiated listeners a better understanding of your concepts.

> *According to most studies, people's number one fear is public speaking. Number two is death. Death is number two. Does that sound right? This means to the average person, if you go to a funeral, you're better off in the casket than doing the eulogy.*
>
> —Jerry Seinfeld

Legal Documents
You Should Have . . . Just in Case

Even thinking about it makes you feel like a total pessimist. You hate planning for the worst; you even think it might jinx you for the future! But it's important to protect yourself in the off-chance that something terrible might actually happen to you. You never expect it, so it is best just to suck it up and sign those key documents that will keep you and your loved ones safe.

Prenup. The last thing you want to think about when you're planning a wedding is divorce, but the truth is that people do change sometimes. If you have assets that need protecting, then protect them! Talk honestly about your finances with your fiancé, and come to a mutual agreement on what's important to you. Having a prenup does not mean you plan to divorce the guy down the road, but should the worst happen, you'll be glad you thought ahead.

Insurance. Homeowners aren't the only ones who need insurance for their property. Renters should sign up for renter's insurance as well! The only thing worse than losing all your property in a fire or flood would be not being able to replace those things you could have if you had bought the insurance to cover them.

194

Living will. This is probably the one document we're most afraid of completing. You feel like you're going to die in a wreck driving home from the lawyer's office! But if you have dependents, you definitely need to sign a will to help them negotiate the legal obstacle course they'll have to travel in those cloudy days of grief. This is one of the best gifts you can give your family—taking care of them after you're gone. (You should also sign a durable power of attorney and a health-care power of attorney when you do your will.) And please, please shell out the extra cash to have a lawyer do this for you; don't buy one of those ready-made wills online.

Birth certificate and Social Security card. You know you have these documents . . . somewhere. Maybe your mom still has them. Or are they in the lockbox at the bank? You'll check on that someday. Many government services require your Social Security card—not just the number, the actual card—before you can take part in the program. And you need your birth certificate to get certain jobs, a passport, and other important documents. So keep these in a safe place and know how to get them quickly. You can go to www.cdc.gov/nchs/howto/w2w/w2welcom.htm to find out how to get a replacement birth certificate, and you can get a replacement Social Security card at www.ssa.gov/ssnumber.

Passport. You may not have that cruise to the Greek isles booked quite yet, but it's still helpful to have a passport nearby just in case. You never know when your boss might want you to join the team on the trip to the London offices—next week. And your passport will suffice for an ID in place of your birth certificate or Social Security card in some instances. You can get the necessary forms to apply for a passport at www.usps.com/passport.

Ways to Be Prepared

for an Emergency—or How to Think Like Dwight Schrute

Know your stuff. You need to create a disaster plan for your family and know what the plans are at your office and your kids' schools. You need to pick two places to meet—one right outside your home and another somewhere in town if you aren't able to get back to your home during the emergency. Choose an out-of-town friend to be a "family contact," because it's usually easier to call long distance in an emergency than it is to call locally. You need to put this number in your cell phone with the letters ICE before it—In Case of Emergency. Emergency workers will be able to quickly identify this as your contact if they find you unconscious after an accident.

Practice your plan. When disaster strikes, it's important to keep a clear head. You don't want your kids running around screaming when the kitchen catches fire—you want them calm, cool, and collected. So practice your emergency plan with them every six months or so. Replace your stored water and food so it's fresh. Test your smoke detectors and fire extinguishers. And if you don't have kids, you can enjoy cracking up at your boyfriend or roommates stumbling in the dark during your surprise fire drill.

Make it obvious. If a meteor crashes through your dining room, you won't have time to go digging for phone numbers and fire extinguishers. You need important info in an obvious place in your house that everyone can find. Post emergency telephone numbers by phones and make sure any kids know *how and when* to call 911. Learn how to turn off water, electricity, and gas to your

196

apartment—you can't waste time flipping through a manual. Make sure you have the right insurance. Know how to use your fire extinguisher, and keep the batteries fresh in the smoke alarms. And identify a "safe place" in your home in case of tornado or earthquake.

Have an emergency kit. You need to put together a box of things you'd need in case of an emergency. Don't procrastinate on this—you'll be really glad you have fresh drinking water if you find yourself stuck at home with no running water or electricity. Here's what to include: one gallon of water per person, three-day supply of nonperishable food, battery-powered radio, flashlight, first-aid kit, a whistle, soap, dust masks for everyone, wet wipes, garbage bags, duct tape, and a tool set (include a can opener for any canned food). If you want more info on things you could pack, log on to the Ready America Web site (www.ready.gov) for a full checklist.[8]

Recovery. Once the actual disaster has passed, there will be a lot you'll have to do to get your life back to normal again. You need to keep your safety and health (physical and mental!) in the front of your mind all the time. If anyone with you is injured, helping them is a top priority. Don't try to move anyone who's seriously hurt— you may just make things worse. However, if you don't have an option, you need to stabilize her neck and back first. Use blankets to keep her warm, and keep everyone's hands clean with soap and water. Don't get yourself overtired—you'll be in "save the world" mode, and the last thing you need is to suffer from exhaustion. Make sure you drink and eat. And be aware of safety concerns around you. You can check out more details about CPR on pages 184–85 and self-defense basics on pages 208–9.

"Your pencils are creating a health hazard. I could fall and pierce an organ."

—Dwight to Jim, *The Office*

Things to Be Sure
to Pack in Your Carry-on Bag

Inevitably, the last thing you think to pack when you're heading out on vacation is the stuff you'll need while you're actually traveling. You're more focused on what you'll wear and use when you get to your destination. But remembering these things will make you feel as if your vacation has already started—before you even get there.

Something to read. How often in your regular life do you have an excuse to do nothing but read or listen to music? What a rare pleasure! Make the most of it. Read the classic you've been dying to get to, indulge yourself with chick lit, or catch up on your favorite magazine from cover to cover. Load your iPod before the trip with your favorite travel songs and all the ones you haven't had a chance to listen to yet.

A change of clothes. You know the feeling of dread that hits your stomach like a ton of bricks when the luggage carousel is empty and your bags have not made the trip around. Your bags have been lost. Having extra undies and a spare outfit in your carry-on takes up very little space and can make a world of difference if something so unfortunate should happen.

Healthy snacks. To keep your energy and morale up while traveling, keep a snack and drink at hand. But make sure it's healthy. Food and drinks loaded with too much sugar, caffeine, preservatives, or unnatural ingredients, added to the circulating stale air and your lack of movement while traveling, will only make you feel dehydrated and more tired.

Directions. Nothing is more frustrating and stressful than getting lost, not knowing exactly where you are, and wasting precious time trying to find your way. Clear, accurate directions or a detailed map can prevent any of the above from taking place—unless you're one of those people who can't read a map or directions! In that case you may want to invest in OnStar or a GPS system for your car.

Medicine. You have the medicine cabinet stocked at home, so why not be prepared for any emergency, or general ache, pain, or unpleasant feelings you may experience when traveling? It only takes one miserably sick passenger to take the fun out of traveling for everyone else.

Questions to Ask
Before You Take the Job

You want this job really badly—or, at least, you *think* you do. It looks perfect on paper: great location, great starting pay, well-known and established company. But all that glitters isn't gold, and it's possible that this dream job could be a nightmare. So don't hesitate to interview your interviewer—ask her some questions that could save you months of agony in the long run.

What do you expect of me? Will your boss expect you to be sitting at your desk from 8:00 to 5:00 with an hour (and no more) for lunch? Or is he more of the mentality that *as long as you get your work done, I don't care when or where you do it*? Were you thinking you might be away from home on business trips once a quarter, and he was thinking once a week? Make sure these expectations are clearly communicated before you start.

What's in it for me? A company has a lot to offer you besides just your paycheck. Many companies have great benefits packages, ranging from great health-care premiums to more unusual perks. For example, Timberland gives its employees $3,000 toward the purchase of a hybrid car. If you're pregnant and work at Eli Lilly, you get the whole month before your due date as paid time off! And J. M. Smucker's employees have no excuse for skipping school—the company offers 100 percent reimbursement for tuition expenses . . . with no limit.[9]

Are you leaving me? If you're not head-over-designer-heels about the position you're taking but you absolutely love the boss you're going to be working for, find out how long he plans to be in his current role. It would be really annoying to be there a month only to find out he's moving over to another department (a promotion that's been in the works for a while) and you won't be working with him again.

Is this a new position? It's helpful to know whether the job you're interviewing for is a new role or if you're replacing someone in an already-existing position. When a company creates a new position, there will be a bigger learning curve for everyone, but there are no comparisons for your coworkers to make between you and the last guy who held your job. If it's an existing job, you'll have a few months to blame all the hiccups on the old guy, but you may have to overcome some bad habits that have become ingrained with him.

Who can I talk to? If the job you're interested in filling is a current position—one where you'll be replacing someone—ask to speak with her about the job. Find out what she loves and what she hates about it. If she's unavailable to speak with you or it's a totally new job you're looking at, find out if there is someone else in a similar position you could speak with. Having an inside scoop will help you confirm your gut instinct about working there.

E-mail Etiquette
Blunders to Avoid

The annoying forwarder. As cute as the pictures of cuddly puppies are, or as funny as the ob-gyn jokes may be, not everyone likes to receive e-mail forwards. In fact, it's probably safe to say that most of us find them really, really annoying. So, before you pass the latest inspirational message on to "ten of your friends" with the promise of blessings, a guilt trip, or even the threat of a curse, carefully evaluate whether they would want to receive it or not. And if the e-mail warns you of a hoax or crime scheme of some sort, check it out on Snopes.com before you send it, just to make sure it's true.

AVOID ALL CAPS. You don't like being yelled at in real life, so why would you like it in e-mail? Not only is writing in all capital letters harder to read, but it comes across as aggressive and pushy. As a general rule, don't use them. Save them for the moments when you're making a point, emphasizing your excitement, or conveying a punch line.

Attachments. When *replying* to an e-mail, you should always attach the prior message. A surprising number of people don't do this. It's frustrating to get an e-mail that says, "Yeah, sounds great" with no other info included. You have no idea what you suggested, and now you have to dig through your sent e-mails to figure out what sounds so great. But when *forwarding* an e-mail, careful thought needs to go into whether to attach the prior message or not! Take the time to evaluate whether the person you are forwarding the e-mail to has the right to, or needs to, see all or part of the previous e-mail.

Did it go through? Be prompt in replying to e-mails, especially in business. Have a policy of replying within twenty-four hours. That way the person on the other end isn't wondering if it went through, debating whether to call you or not. And if you're going to be away from your computer for a while, put an automatic response up so others will know you're not checking e-mails for a while.

Double-check what you're sending before you hit Send. Have you ever checked your e-mail only to discover a batch of quite personal photos—a friend's *very* pregnant belly and her husband cuddling it or documentation of your coworker's weekend away with her boyfriend? A second e-mail probably quickly came —*I attached the wrong photos! Please delete!* Make sure you're sending what you mean to send by double-checking all your attachments and info.

"People will now e-mail someone across the room rather than go and talk to them. But I don't think this is laziness, I think it is a conscious decision people are making to save time."[10]

—Margaret J. Wheatley

Ways to Say,
"I'm Sorry."

The business apology. In business the customer or client is always right. It doesn't matter if you're certain that you turned in the order the way *they* placed it or you *did* in fact tell them the interest rate would apply to their contract. If they say you screwed up, and you want to keep their business, you apologize for the misunderstanding and promise that the situation will be resolved quickly. But it's also appropriate for you to let your boss know that you're not at fault if you have the documentation showing you aren't actually in the wrong. Just be quick to reassure him that you are more than happy to take the blame and rectify the problem to help the company.

The family apology. If your sister has ever stood you up at your birthday dinner, or your mom has ever divulged your darkest secret to all your aunts (who spread it to the rest of the family, and so on), you know that family feuds can be incredibly frustrating, hurtful, and complicated. But your family is not going to disappear, no matter how offended you are. You can't just write them off and walk away as if you never knew them. So when you're the one in the wrong, be quick to offer a sincere apology. Don't make excuses. Just acknowledge that you were inconsiderate and foolish, and you want to do what it takes to make things right.

The major offense apology. Sometimes a simple "I'm sorry" is not going to cut it. If you've genuinely screwed up—done something bordering on unforgivable—it will require an apology proportional to the crime. This apology must be done in person, with plenty of time set aside to talk things through.

Be honest. Do not excuse your behavior. Admit that you are wrong. And look her in the eyes when you ask for forgiveness. Assure her that you want to make the situation better, and ask what you can do to convince her of your willingness to resolve the situation. Understand if it takes her awhile to forgive and forget.

The bigger-person apology. When it comes down to it, you realize that both you and your boyfriend are wrong. He was a jerk in demanding that you stay home with him instead of going out with the girls, and you were a jerk to ditch him without as much as a text message when you went out with them anyway. But you realize that the relationship is more important to you than being "right." Tell him you're sorry you hurt him by leaving him out in the cold, but that you were hurt as well. Admitting your fault will open the door to an apology from him as well.

The I-still-don't-really-think-it's-that-big-of-a-deal apology.
Sometimes you just don't get what the big deal is. Your coworker is freaking out that you didn't call her when you came to town for a meeting, but you're really not that close with her and would never have expected her to do the same for you. When you can't imagine what's gotten another person so upset, it's hard to make a genuine apology. But if the tension is making life annoying, offer a warm and affectionate "I'm sorry." You may need to have a follow-up conversation with the person to establish realistic expectations for the relationship.

Things You Need to Know

to Defend Yourself from an Attacker

Know what's going on around you. You know the feeling you get when something bad is about to happen—your boyfriend is about to dump you, your least-favorite person has just pulled in the driveway, or a strange man is acting weird in the parking lot. Your heart pounds a little harder. You start to sweat just a bit. And you can feel the anxiety growing. Trust that instinct. Pay attention to people who seem to stare too long, follow you too closely, or pass by you more than one time. They may be checking you out to see how you'll react if they try to attack. Let them know you're not going to be passive—look them in the eye; let them see your strength.

A woman is like a tea bag. You never know how strong she is until she gets into hot water.

—Eleanor Roosevelt

People are key. Do your best to make sure an attacker does not get you alone anywhere. If other people are around, your chances of escaping unscathed are much higher. So don't get in the car. Don't go into an alley. Scream for help. Climb out the window. Blow the horn. Drive your car to a restaurant parking lot. Throw something. He may threaten you, but you're much less likely to survive if you're alone in the woods with him.

206

Don't make it easy for him. You want to make it as hard as possible for him to get to you. So no matter what he says, don't help him attack you. Don't unlock the door for him. Spray pepper spray or mace. Force him to work hard to get to you. According to Defend University, a self-defense school, "The more difficult you make it, the more time it takes him and that means he might be discovered."[11]

> To learn more specific self-defense moves, visit Defend University's website at www.defendu.com. You can sign up for classes or buy a self-defense DVD.

Control him. Put your feet on his hips— your legs are very strong and will be your best protection against rape. And his hands are what will do the damage in slapping, hitting, or worse—stabbing—you. So block any movements with your forearms; or better yet, take his arms out of commission. If you have anything you can use to break his arm, don't hesitate. You'll need to enroll in a self-defense course to learn how to keep an attacker's body off of yours. This is one of the best things you can do for yourself, so sign up today.

Use your strength against his weakness. Your legs and elbows are the strongest parts of your body, and hammer-fist moves and strikes with the heel of your palm are very effective. So what should you target with these blows? His weak but valuable body parts—eyes, throat, crotch, knees, nose, and stomach. Go crazy on him—kick and hit until you can kick and hit no more. Show no mercy.

notes

Part One
Social Butterfly: Relationsip Essentials

1. Marilyn Ellis, "A Laugh a Day May Help Keep Death Further Away," *USA Today*, http://www.usatoday.com/news/health/2007-03-11-health-laughter_N.htm.
2. Saul Hansell, "For MySpace, Making Friends Was Easy. Big Profit is Tougher," NY *Times*, http://www.nytimes.com/2006/04/23/business/yourmoney/23myspace.html?ei=5088&en=68144371c2be06ac&ex=1303444800&pagewanted=all.
3. Wendy Norlund, "Why We Laugh and Cry," http://www.gibbsmagazine.com/CryinLaughing.htm.
4. Ana Marie Cox, "Can New Hampshire Revive McCain?," *Time*, http://www.time.com/time/politics/article/0,8599,1661275,00.html.
5. Bill Cosby, *Love and Marriage* (New York: Bantom, a division of Random House, 1990).
6. Thomas Perls, *Living to 100* (New York: Basic, 2000). www.livingto100.com.
7. 3 John 1:4 KJV
8. The information in this section comes from http://elementaltruths.blogspot.com/2006/08/12-ways-to-win argument.html.
9. See Chapman, Gary, *The Five Love Languages* (Chicago: Northfield Publishers, 1995).

Part Two
Classy and Fabulous: Lifestyle Essentials

1. Carey McBeth-Cooper is owner of Essential Etiquette, Mastering the Art of Good Manners based in Vancouver, Canada. 604-317-3299.
2. David Adam, "Circle Me, Lord," www.worldprayers.org (accessed on February 26, 2007).
3. Mechthild of Magdeburg, "Lord, you are my lover," www.worldprayers.org (accessed on February 26, 2007).
4. Dame Julian of Norwich, "All shall be well," www.worldprayers.org (accessed on February 26, 2007).
5. Matthew 6:9–13, NRSV
6. From *Lanterns: A Memoir of Mentors* by Marian Wright Edelman. Copyright © 1999 by Marian Wright Edelman. Reprinted by permission of Beacon Press, Boston.
7. Thanks to Heidi LaFleche for the term "cubicle lurkers." http://content.monster.com/articles/3488/17862/1/default.aspx.
8. Kate Lorenz, "10 Ways to Maintain Your Privacy at Work," Career Builder, http://www.careerbuilder.com/JobSeeker/careerbytes/CBArticle.aspx?articleID=490&cbRecursionCnt=3&cbsid=ffa01c5f13f943b7a442201926ff4fd8-232457861-VH-4.
9. *Helicobacter pylori* and Peptic Ulcer Disease Myths," Centers for Disease Control and Prevention, http://www.cdc.gov/ulcer/myth.htm.

Notes

10. Much thanks to Dan Briody for his hilarious thoughts on cell phone usage. For more see Dan Briody, "The Ten Commandments of Cell Phone Etiquette," Infoworld, http://www.infoworld.com/articles/op/xml/00/05/26/000526opwireless.html (accessed March 5, 2007).
11. Joanna L. Krotz, "Cell Phone Etiquette: 10 Dos and Don'ts," Microsoft Small Business Center, http://www.microsoft.com/smallbusiness/resources/technology/communications/cell_phone_etiquette_10_dos_and_donts.mspx (accessed March 5, 2007).
12. The information in this article is paraphrased from http://interiordesign.lovetoknow.com/Bargaining_Tips_for_Flea_Market_and_Antique_Shopping.
13. "Why Aren't You Supposed to Wear White After Labor Day?" http://ask.yahoo.com/20020913.html.
14. Our thanks to Dr. Paul J. Rosch, President of the American Institute of Stress, for his direction and advice in this chapter.
15. Liz Pulliam Weston, "The Truth About Credit Card Debt," MSN, http://moneycentral.msn.com/content/Banking/creditcardsmarts/P74808.asp.

Part Three
Domestic Goddess: Home Essentials

1. Visit http://www.foodnetwork.com/food/recipes/recipe/0,1977,FOOD_9936_19793,00.html for the full recipe.
2. Some of the info here is from Randy Cassingham, "Help with Spam and Phishing," http://www.spamprimer.com/2-nowwhat.html.
3. Special thanks to Susan Kelton, http://associates.era.com/susankelton, for her advice on this section.
4. Info sourced from "MacGyver Tip: Dishwashing liquid ice pack," LifeHacker.com, http://lifehacker.com/sofware/macgyver/macgyver-tip-dishwashing-liquid-ice-pack-151727.php.
5. All members of the Pet Sitter's Association, LLC are covered by General Liability Insurance for their pet-sitting business.
6. Special thanks to Susan Kelton, http://associates.era.com/susankelton, for her advice on this section.
7. Info sourced from Renu Dalal-Jain, "Five Simple Ways to Organize Your Closet Today," GotLinks.com, http://www.gotlinks.com/earticles/articles/69715-five-simple-ways-to-organize-your-closet-today_.html.
8. The ideas here come from http://www.rentaldecorating.com/0406/ten_tips_for_small_spaces.htm and http://interiordec.about.com/od/articlesonbasics/a/smallroomtricks.htm.
9. Sourced from Paul McKenzie, "Easier Gardening," HGTV.com, http://www.hgtv.com/hgtv/gl_gardening_basics/article/0,1785,HGTV_3589_3877445,00.html.

Part Four
Fetching and Fit: Body Essentials

1. "Folic Acid," March of Dimes, www.marchofdimes.com/pnhec/173_769.asp.
2. Dr. Dan Rutherford, "Sources of Minerals," NetDoctor, www.netdoctor.com.uk/focus/nutrition/facts/vitamins_minerals.htm.
3. www.brainyquote.com/quotes/quotes/h/hulkhogan198770.html.
4. Dr. Dan Rutherford, "Sources of Minerals."
5. "Vitamins," TeensHealth, www.kidshealth.org/teen/misc/vitamin_chart.html.
6. Daniel J. DeNoon, "Dark Chocolate is Healthy Chocolate," WebMD, www.webmd.com/diet/news/20030827/dark-chocolate-is-healthy-chocolate.
7. Shiela Dicks, "Beauty Tips for Luscious Lips," Ezine articles, http://ezinearticles.com/?beatuy-Tips-for-luscious-Lips&id:15585.
8. Preventing Heart Disease: What Women Need to Know," American College of Cardiology. www.acc.org.
9. Richard Carlson, Don't Sweat the Small Stuff (New York: Hyperion, 1999). www.dontsweat.com.
10. "Exercise Reduces Stress," University of Iowa Hospitals and Clinics, www.unihealthcare.com.

Notes

11. Melina B. Jampolis, MD, *No Time to Lose Diet* (Nashville: Thomas Nelson, 2006).
12. Check them out online at www.whfoods.org.
13. Meline B. Jampolis, *No Time to Lose Diet*, 40, 44–45, 46, 49–50.
14. The specific link to this list is found at www.childbirth.org/articles/remedy.html.
15. "12 Tips to Treat Colds and Flu the'Natural' Way," WebMd, www.webmd.com/cold-and-flu/12-natural-treatments-for-the-flu.
16. "50 Ways to Fight Cold and Flu," LocateaDoc.com, www.locateadoc.om/article.cfm/search/93.

Part Five
Does It All: All the Other Essentials

1. "Study: Using Big Words Needlessly Makes You Seem Stupider," Collision Detection, http://www.collisiondetection .net/mt/archives/2006/04/study_using_big.html.
2. Paraphrased from Theryn Fleming, "10 Quick Fixes That'll Make You Look Really Smart . . . or How *Not* to Peeve an Editor," http://www.toasted-cheese.com/ab/02-08.htm.
3. Ibid.
4. Proverbs 17:28 NIV
5. The information in this section comes from "Car/Auto Mechanics: Putting a Dent in Your Wallet," Service Snitch, http://www.servicesnitch.com/site/article/car_auto_mechanics_putting_a_dent_in_your_wallet/.
6. "Learn CPR: You Can Do It," http://depts.washington.edu/learncpr/quickcpr.html.
7. The information in this section comes from Trent Hamm, "25 Things You Should Always Have in Your Car," The Simple Dollar, http://www.thesimpledollar.com/2007/03/18/25-things-you-should-always-have-in-your-car/.
8. The Full website link is www.ready.gov/american/getakit/index.html.
9. Fortune 100 Best Companies to Work For, "Unusual Perks," CNNMoney.com, http://money.cnn.com/magazines/fortune/bestcompanies/best_benefits/unusual.html.
10. Margaret J. Wheatley, "Is the Pace of Life Hindering Our Ability to Manage?" *Management Today*, March 2004.
11. "Self-defense Principles," Defend University, http://www.defendu.com/wsdi/principles.htm.